Love Myself Slim

Love Myself Slim

*Learning to love yourself & lose weight.
Understanding & changing the childhood
patterns which trap you in low
self-esteem & over-eating*

Jonathan Whines

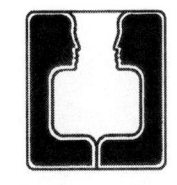

**Dialogue Press
London 2010**

Published by:
Dialogue Press
www.dialogueconsultancy.com

© 2010 by Jonathan Whines

All rights reserved. No part of this book may be reproduced in any form or by any means, electronic or mechanical, including photocopying, recording or by any information storage and retrieval system, without permission in writing from the publisher.

First Edition

Printed in The United Kingdom

Contents

Preface

Chapter One	Understanding the Body-Mind Dis-Connect	1
Chapter Two	The Blueprint of Your Emotional Life "Rules are not Truths"	15
Chapter Three	How We Learn to Bury Our Feelings	58
Chapter Four	Avoiding Feelings & Over-Eating	84
Chapter Five	These Emotions Are Nothing to do with Me	99
Chapter Six	This Body is Nothing to do with Me Either	116
Chapter Seven	Shame	127
Chapter Eight	Food, Eating & the Development of Identity	148
Chapter Nine	Mindfulness & Over-Eating	156
Chapter Ten	Compassion & Self-Easteem	179
Chapter Eleven	The Renewal & Recovery Programme	195
Appendix 1	Full Exercise Listing	204
Bibliography & Resources		217
Glossary		220

Acknowledgements

Developing as a psychotherapist and a writer takes a lot of work and training. It also requires that many people give of their time and energy to support you. I am indebted to many trainers and teachers on my own journey. These include all the Gestalt staff at the Metanoia Institute in London epecially, Jenny Mackewn and Talia Levine Bar-Joseph. Trainers at Bangor University Centre for Mindfulness particularly Judith Soulsby and to John Crook, an inspiring Zen teacher.

Thanks to my superviser Phil Joyce for his generous support and to my partner Jacqui Hughes for her love and support. Finally, my greatest learning has occured through working with my clients. Thankyou to all of you for sharing your stories and lives with me.

Preface

People come in all shapes and sizes so feeling good about yourself is more important than demanding that you have to be slim. However, if you want to lose weight it will help considerably if you understand some of the psychological issues that may prevent this.

This book will encourage and challenge you to consider how you feel about food, your feelings and yourself. At the heart of this approach is the development of a mindful and compassionate attitude towards yourself - so we would encourage you to try and adopt this attitude of kindness from the beginning.

When we over-eat it is often because we feel sad or angry or our self-esteem is low. Try to cultivate a loving attitude towards yourself as you travel along this new path of discovery. As a first step buy yourself a journal and following the exercises start to keep a record of this journey.

June 2010

Chapter One

Understanding The Body-Mind Disconnect

Introduction

Thousands of diet books proclaim the virtues of eating according to certain plans. They encourage more of this food less of that. They all meet with a degree of success and a degree of failure. What they miss is that the ideas in their books will encounter a particular mind-set. When it comes to food most of us have quite powerful attitudes learnt when we were young. The ideas in the diet books are bit like firing arrows at a well-defended castle. Most of us are psychologically not so different to the castle. So, however good the concepts are we often fail at dieting because we do not understand our own psychology and the patterns learnt from the past which keep us over-eating.

At the heart of most abusive behaviour and over-eating is a form of abuse, lies a fundamental loss of compassion. This may manifest as a loss of compassion for the world but is more truly a loss of compassion for ourselves.

How and why we lose compassion for ourselves is a compelling and usually sad story. How we regain compassion requires a careful de-construction and reconstruction of our inner world.

The Body-Mind Dis-Connect

To be compassionate requires a clear understanding of the guiding principles or introjects we were taught as children. These numerous overt and implied rules created the internal emotional structure of who we were to become. These "rules" which created us, need our focussed attention, for they are often hidden or clouded by their very ordinariness. It is only as we start to discriminate the usefulness or otherwise of these rules that we can start to discover who we really are.

So, the primary goal of this book is to develop a more compassionate sense of who we are. One of the benefits of this will be our ability to regulate our emotions more effectively, connect with our body and therefore to develop a healthier relationship with food and eating.

We will explore how we came to lose our compassion in the first place: how we lost our ability to like and love ourselves in our being and only give credit for what we do or achieve. We will explore key psychological patterns or what I call the "emotional blueprint" which leads us into over-eating. In conjunction with exploring the psychology of over-eating we will also incorporate exercises in mindfulness to help you develop a greater awareness of yourself. You will be encouraged to explore your sensations, emotions and needs and how, when you over-eat, you constantly interrupt the meeting of these most essential needs.

How I eat and relate to food is intimately connected to how I manage my emotional life. The key issues in this regard are

- Was I brought up to believe that I am a separate and autonomous person with a right to my own ideas and beliefs ie was my individuality and uniqueness as a person respected?

- Was I taught to value and express my feelings, thoughts and needs? Was I taught to be assertive and meet my needs?

The Body-Mind Dis-Connect

The reason this book is called *Love Myself Slim* is because under-pinning all of the above issues is one central question:

- Did I feel loved and lovable, in my uniqueness and could I express my love to others?

In my experience many clients who have weight issues usually answer "no" to at least one of the three questions and always answer "no" the last question.

How do I start to find myself lovable whilst also believing it is fine to be different, unique, expressive, assertive and meet my needs. These are usually the major issues for clients with weight issues.

Love Myself Slim then sets out to explore in detail all the many and varied ruptures which occur to our sense of being loved and lovable. Further, it describes the breaks and breaches in this love-circuit and then offers exercises and meditations to start to repair this loss of love. It is only when we can genuinely start to feel more loved and lovable, in our uniqueness, that we will be able to stop "self-medicating" this sense of emptiness by over-eating. When we feel good about ourselves food just becomes... food, rather than an endless comforter covering up our yearning and longing for "something else".

How To Use This Book

People read and learn in different ways. We also all have very different needs. I would encourage you to read this book in the way that works for you. Most of the chapters can be read independently. If you find something that interests you it is fine to dip in, read the theoretical part and then try the exercises.

The Body-Mind Dis-Connect

Generally speaking we usually tend to be more blocked in one aspect of our psychology than another. You may therefore find yourself more drawn to exploring certain elements of yourself.

However, the system presented here is highly interconnected and the total book represents this. Therefore, you may find that as you work through one part of yourself another element of your psychology comes more to the fore. It may be that you will then want to explore more deeply in the book.

I have suggested you be guided by your own interest in how you read the book yet also notice if you feel pushed away by certain topics. It may be this area is the very chapter you really need to read! Try to approach what you read with an openness to exploring. From hundreds of hours working with clients I know that these exercises, when fully engaged with, can have a profound and life-changing effect.

Equally, if you like to read a book cover to cover that is fine. Just make sure you go slowly enough to really engage with the exercises. Although some of the methods may initially seem artificial – such as writing a letter expressing your feeling to someone who has left you or who has died – they can elicit very powerful emotions. So, always make some quiet time to engage with the exercises and ensure you have enough space after an exercise so you do not have to rush back into the busyness of your life!

The Body-Mind Dis-Connect

Creating a Programme

As you travel through the book in whatever way works for you note the exercises which impact on you or support you more than others. Become used to the idea of challenging the old rules by which you have lived and learn the many new ways to support yourself found throughout the book. As you do so build this into your own personal programme. I will discuss your personal programme in more detail at the end of the book. Try to get in the habit of writing down your responses to the exercises. Pay particular attention to what you find supportive and commit to turning these small moments of support into a new you.

Over the years I have come to some foundational conclusions about why we over-eat. You may agree or you may find these ideas difficult. I would simply ask that you keep an open-mind and try exploring the ideas and exercises which follow.

Key ideas 1 & 2:

1. **We over-eat because we want to avoid how we feel about other people & the world.**

2. **We over-eat because we want to avoid how we feel about ourselves**

Exercise 1.1: Body & Emotions

- If you are unclear about the relationship between your emotions and your body try the following exercise. Firstly close your eyes:

The Body-Mind Dis-Connect

- Think and or picture something or someone you love. What happens in your body. What physical sensations do you experience? Does your body feel warm, cold, relaxed etc.

- Think and or picture something or someone you dislike. What happens in your body? What sensations do you experience and where? Do you shoulders become tense or do you feel a knot in your stomach.

You may experience a warmth or opening sensation in part one and a tightening or closing in part two. This process of opening and closing is happening all the time, everyday in us as we experience the world. It is simply that we have often been taught to filter it out. Re-connecting with this process will help you to start to regain control of your emotional life.

Compassion

Young mothers and fathers generally set out with a deep sense of love and caring for their children yet somewhere along the developmental path this love and sense of compassion can get partially obscured or even lost. The loving parent becomes critical, judgemental, aggressive, passive, demanding of attention or demanding that the identity of the child should conform only to their wishes.

Parents are not generally bad but rather they play out the patterns of the parenting to which they were exposed. The loss of compassion in the parent becomes reflected in the child in the imposition of rules at the expense of encouraging the child to listen to the wisdom and needs of their own body

The Body-Mind Dis-Connect

To understand why we might have learnt to disconnect from our bodies we need to appreciate how our identity is formed in the first place:

Identity & Contact

Our identity develops primarily through the contact we have with our parents. The emotional tone of our up-bringing plus the rules we are taught and shown forms to a large degree who we are.

Jessica's mother was passive and caring she never put herself first, her father by contrast was domineering and bullying. Jessica related more to her mother so she learnt to be caring and passive but also she took on her fathers attitude and bullied herself – never feeling she was enough or could live up to his expectations. The family generally did not express or talk about their emotions. Jessica learnt to disconnect from her body and that her needs were unimportant.

Jessica became a nurse which suited her caring nature. She had a boss who was highly organised and so she constantly felt that she could not live up to her bosses expectations. Whilst her boss thought Jessica was doing fine Jessica would constantly over-work but did not feel she could express her anxieties and stress.

When she went home Jessica would often start to over-eat. She was aware of feeling "a bit empty" which was:

"a bit like feeling hungry, plus" .

Apart from this she did not really feel anything else at all. After she had eaten she would then criticize herself , vow to do better but then continue to over-eat because she felt so un-happy with herself regarding her eating. Jessica was trapped in a self-destructive loop.

Diet & Blocking the Sensation our Feelings

"All feelings start with sensation. If we do not know what is happening in our body we cannot know what we feel emotionally"

At the heart of Jessica's problem she has learnt through her up-bringing to disconnect from her body. This has a number of effects:

- She is unaware of the sensations in her body. She was taught from an early age to not listen to her body and to priorititise the needs of others.

- Because she is unaware of her sensation she is also disconnected from how she feels because all emotion originates in sensation – the tightening of your chest, the knot in your belly is the beginning of sadness or fear.

- Even if she has some idea of how she feels it won't be acceptable because her feelings will bring her into conflict with others. Conflict is out of the question for Jessica because it reminds her of her father and that in the end she will come off worst in a conflict or she will, even worse, become like her father.

Disconnected from her body and her sensation she won't know what her feelings are. Disconnected from her emotions she won't know what she needs.

The Body-Mind Dis-Connect

The ever changing pattern of our needs are in part who we are. Not knowing what our needs are means we do not really know who we are. Disconnected from our bodies we are fundamentally disconnected from the essence of who we are. Jessica therefore exists in a fog of half-known feelings and half-known needs which she cannot truly satisfy. Her only comfort for this strange "hunger" is to fill the vacuum by over-eating

Key Ideas: 3

Unexpressed emotion or thought can be experienced as a numbness, emptyness or a generalised sense of dis-satisfaction. This "hunger" can be appeased by dealing with the emotional issues or by avoiding the emotions. A primary method of avoiding emotion is to over-eat.

Re-Connect with your Body

In order for Jessica to re-connect with her body and understand what she is feeling she needs to become more aware of the sensations in her body. She needs to both get to know and to re-inhabit her own body. To start this journey she needs to develop a more conscious, mindful experience of her body

If you feel unfamiliar with the idea of noticing your bodily sensations then take the following exercise slowly in 2 parts:

Firstly, just observe and notice sensations. Once you feel comfortable with this move to the second part to see if you can associate feelings with these sensations.

Exercise.1.2: Zones

Imagine dividing your body into 10 zones.

1. Brow & crown of your head
2. Eyes & temples
3. Mouth & Jaw
4. Throat
5. Arms, shoulders & hands
6. Chest, heart & solar plexus
7. Belly
8. Genitals
9. Legs
10. Feet

- Breathing slowly, move your attention or **awareness** carefully through these ten zones.
- Be aware of what **sensations** you find in each zone
- Name the sensation ie tight, hot, cold, relaxed, like a spring
- Once you've identified a sensation **give this sensation a voice** ie "My leg feels tight like it wants to kick something"

The Body-Mind Dis-Connect

- Try to **identify the emotion** you connect with the sensation

- "My tight leg feels angry"

- **Try to explore who this anger might be aimed at**: your partner, a friend, your boss, yourself. "Who do I want to kick!"

- Initially simply allow yourself to be aware of the emotion

Staying with Jessica we might imagine as she does this exercise she becomes aware of a tightly coiled spring in her chest –she identifies this as a mixture of anxiety and anger with her boss. Anxious that she feels her boss is very demanding and angry because her boss is so perfect. She then realises she is also angry with herself because she does not feel perfect.

To recap then:

- Slow yourself down by breathing deeply and slowly

- Track through the 10 zones

- Notice any sensations

- When you find a sensation be curious if there is any emotion or image attached to the sensation.

- Check if the emotion is directed at others or yourself

- Find a way to express this emotion which is "safe enough" for you

The Body-Mind Dis-Connect

For example, I might feel tight in my throat, I feel slightly choked, I wonder, what or who is choking me? Further, what emotions do I associate with choking: anxiety and anger. I have a picture of my boss with his hands round my throat. If I'm Jessica I might think "You are choking the life out of me with your demands". See the diagram on the next page.

The Cycle of Awareness

Our body-mind when functioning naturally, as with a young child, is constantly moving through the cycle described on the left side of the diagram. We call this the Cycle of Awareness. Sensations and emotions arise, are expressed in the form of needs, action is taken, if required and the issue is closed. A baby experiences dryness in her mouth, this unpleasant sensation constellates as thirst, the thirst makes her frustrated so she takes action and cries. The mother recognises the cry as a demand for a drink and offers the child some milk or juice. The baby drinks, the liquid resolves the dryness and the issue of being thirsty is closed. The baby smiles ready for the next emerging need!

The Body-Mind Dis-Connect

A flow chart of this process might look like the following:

Breathing
⇩
Sensation
⇩
Awareness
⇩
Emotion or Visual Image
⇩
Choice Point – ie choosing what to do re. feelings
⇩

Expression of Feelings   OR   Suppression
of Feeling
⇩
Action (if required)   Physical/emotional
reaction/symptoms

⇩

CLOSURE   OVER-EATING

Chapter Two

The Blueprint of Your Emotional Life: "Rules are not Truths"

Interrupting The Cycle of Awareness

The Cycle of Awareness which is so important to our emotional and bodily health can be interrupted at all stages in the process. Part of recovering our re-connection is becoming aware of the old patterns which cause us to block the natural flow of our own body-mind process. Lets explore how this can happen.

If you observe a young baby as described above they laugh, cry, demand food and sleep. They are in complete contact with their bodies, sensations and emotions. We might see this as a totally free process which flows without any interruption from their parents or society. Of course as time passes the parents start to encourage certain behaviours more than others. They tell the child off if it cries too much, they praise the child if it eats all its food. Whether spoken or modelled the child starts to realise there are certain rules. Whatever the rules, however good or bad these are the norm for that family. As children we drink these rules in, a bit like liquid, these rules then start to form who we are and how we behave.

Clients who come to see me often do not realise that they are operating out of a whole set of rules which they took on years before. These rules, known as introjects, are a bit like the underlying operating software in a computer –ie certain computer processes just happen without my needing to do anything. In the same way we often react to situations in an automatic way. We are functioning from our old operating system. If the rules are not very good ones this can be detrimental to our health and wellbeing.

It is important to realize:

Key Ideas 4:

What was the norm in your family was not necessarily normal or healthy for you. Understand what rules or operating system you live by. Then, a bit like chewing food we need to chew over the old rules we were given and decide if they actually accord with who we are today.

As we grow as children we necessarily have to be socialised into the ways of the world. However, as this process occurs it often means that we become more detached from the truth of our own sensations and bodies. This detachment from our lived physical experience means we are also not fully in connection with our own unique emotional experience.

Rules about our Body

- Parents may give all sorts of messages about their relationship with their body and how the child should view their own body. I am describing these as "rules" – it is important to understand that these may be explicit and spoken rules or more often they may be behaviours

Rules Are Not Truths

modelled to you within the family which you have taken on over time. Every family is a little tribe and will operate according to certain customs. Understanding these rules or customs will enable you to become clearer about your own thinking and behaviour. The following are some examples:

- "Getting the job done is more important than your body. Ignore your hunger, apply your will and don't think about eating". This attitude often underlies clients who become highly stressed. They may go for years not listening to their body until finally their body fights back and they become ill.

- "Mind is more important than body". People who are academic or intellectual who again simply dis-regard and disconnect from their body.

- "Your body is dangerous –it may lead you into temptation". The body is seen as something that should be controlled or limited as it may cause you to do wild and crazy things like flirting, being sexual, dancing outrageously or playing in a rock n roll band!!

- "Your body is dangerous – you might get angry". Rather than seeing anger as just another emotion it is seen as something unwelcome and dangerous that must again be controlled.

Exercise 2.1: Body Rules

Reflect on your childhood. What sort of attitude did your parents have to their own bodies and what did they teach you about your relationship with your body. If this is a difficult area for you, be compassionate with yourself and explore this carefully. Write down examples of the sort of messages you learnt. Having written them down reflect on whether these are rules that continue to be useful or whether it is time to reject them. Be aware of how difficult or not it is to contradict your parent's view. If you find this hard don't worry as challenging these old rules can be difficult and we will spend a lot of time examining this. For the moment just notice how difficult it is to stand up to your parents view and score that difficulty 1 -10 with 1 being easy and 10 being impossible.

Jessica's father was very strict. He believed in the imposition of his will power over his body and expected the same of Jessica. She therefore learnt to over-work and not be aware of the stress she was placing on her body

Key Ideas 5: When considering what we learnt from our parents it is important to remember that when we reject an idea or a rule we do not need to totally reject them as people. It is simply important to discriminate what is helpful and healthy in your life and what is not. Your parents did the best they could given the parenting they had. Try to discriminate what you need and be compassionate both with yourself and them.

Rules about Food

Because food plays such an important role in the life of a child this is one of the areas where rules of behaviour get learnt very early. Food can be easy or become a battleground where the parent's deepest beliefs get played out. For example:

Rules Are Not Truths

Mother: " I am in complete control. You will eat when and how I demand

Mother:"I allow baby to completely dominate mealtime – I cannot assert myself"

Mother: "I use food to pacify baby when she is irritable"" It doesn't matter if baby sometimes needs to wait to be fed food isn't that important "

In these examples food becomes a powerful instrument of domination or control both ways between mother and baby.

Exercise 2.2: Food Rules

Reflect on your childhood. What sort of attitude did your parents have towards food and what did this teach you about your current relationship with food. Write down examples of the sort of messages you learnt. Having written them down reflect on whether these are rules that continue to be useful or whether it is time to reject them. Again, be aware of how difficult or not it is to contradict your parent's view. If you find this hard don't worry as challenging these old rules can be difficult and we will spend a lot of time examining this. For the moment just notice how difficult it is to stand up to your parents view and score that difficulty 1 -10 with 1 being easy and 10 being impossible

Rules about You

In addition to the "rules" about bodies and food are the rules or customs which apply to you specifically:

Rules Are Not Truths

Family Position

The first consideration is your position in the family. All sorts of expectations will arise out of your position in the family. For example my brother was the oldest child, he experienced needing to be very responsible. He felt that there were lots of expectations placed on him as the older one. I was the youngest of three and experienced a very laissez faire childhood where my parents had relaxed into parenthood, were financially better off and generally more relaxed with me. My sister who was born in the middle felt there was more attention placed on the two boys and therefore, typically for the middle child and especially as a girl, struggled with being seen.

Typical Rules Re. Family Position

The Oldest Child: More will be demanded of you. Your parents are likely to be more anxious as first time parents. They will check your behaviour more. They are likely to be less well-off so will have more generalised anxiety. They may also be more focussed upon their careers as they establish themselves so they may be more "absent" than in later years. Because of issues around anxiety and responsibility these may be considerations for you which underly over-eating as a compensatory mechanism to help you feel better at times of stress.

When the second child is born there may be issues of you feeling your position has been usurped. Negotiating this can be a tricky issue for parents and can often remain un-resolved. Being the Queen/King who lost their crown can be difficult!

Rules Are Not Truths

Rules for the Oldest

Rules for the oldest might include: "You should be the best... as you are the first child representative of this family".... nothing less than a Beckham or a Pavarotti will do, failing that doctor or lawyer will sort of be ok!!"You must be ultra-responsible and not let the family down ... as for above. "Be very careful".... because you are especially precious to us and we don't want you to make a mistake! "You should love your little sister/brother... what when my crown has just been stolen and I had all that love/attention to myself??"

The Middle Child: There will be less demand and anxiety placed upon you. However, middle children often feel that they do not get the attention or indeed the expectations of the first born. There is somehow a struggle for their lives and identity to be as important as the older sibling – a sort of second best quality.

Rules for the Middle Child

Rules for the middle child might include:

"Look up to your brother/sister, do as they say"

"It's all right to be ignored"

""What you do is less important"

The Youngest Child

The youngest child often experiences much less anxiety regarding their up-bringing as their parents are financially and emotionally more secure. They will be much more relaxed about risk taking. The world will generally seem a more benign place than in the early days of parenthood when every step of the child held the potential for disaster! Because of all this the youngest often feels special which can be great and can tip into a narcicisstic sense of self-importance and conceit. Receiving less restriction from their parents and possibly the indulgence of their siblings youngest children often have a sense that the normal rules do not apply. If they are charming they can get just what they want. Equally the youngest can sometimes feel left out and as though they never quite belong with the adults. Not something I know anything about at all!

Rules for the Youngest Child

Some possible rules for the youngest might include

"You can get away with things"

"The earlier rules do not apply"

"People will inevitably like and listen to you"

"Charm can get you anything you want"

"You're the kid, what do you know?"

Only Children

Only children often have a curious mixture of being the oldest and the youngest. They have all the anxiety and responsibility taking of the oldest whilst being the favoured child who has to make no compromise with siblings. In addition there is no escape from attention of their parents and there are no other children to play with so only children often have to develop a powerful internal life in order to maintain a sense of who they are.

Rules for the Only Child

"You are our only special child you hold ALL our hopes" ... no pressure there then!! "You can always have exactly what YOU want because there are no other children you have to compromise with" ... is that a little princess I see coming!!

Exercise 2.3: Family Position

Consider your position in the family what were the rules or assumptions based upon this position? What pressures, anxieties or demands arose simply because of your position in the family? Consider to what degree you were pressured or ignored because of your positioning?

Write down a list of these rules. As you look at the list breathe slowly and become aware of the 10 Zones. Notice what sensations arise as you consider the rules. As the sensations arise try and name what emotions or images you associate with the sensation.

Jessica was the eldest child she felt the burden of responsibility of this in several ways. Her rules would be:

"You must always achieve highly"

"You should put others first and care for them before yourself"

As Jessica breathes and listens to her body she becomes aware of the fury she has with her father for being so demanding and for not really seeing her as a person.

Rules Are Not Truths

Externalising Exercise 2.4:

Expressing Emotion about an Old Rule & Creating a New One

One of the ways which we will work in the book is that we will uncover a rule or introject and then the sensation and emotion which goes with this. We will then use a special exercise to "externalise" the feeling. As described feelings which remain un-concluded will block up our emotional-energetic system. We will become tired and depressed without really knowing why and this, of course, will probably lead to over-eating.

So, reflecting upon the rule and the emotion this generates try to hold a picture of the person who gave you this rule. To fully externalise them imagine they are sitting in a chair opposite you. Find a short sentence which contradicts the rule.

Jessica struggles to say anything to her father as she is both still afraid of him and feels protective of him. With some encouragement that this is just an exercise Jessica eventually says to her imagined father:

1. *" I am angry with you and I am no longer prepared to be bullied and dominated by you"*

Jessica acknowledges her feelings towards her father and for the first time stands up to him. She is then encouraged to make a positive statement of intent regarding the old rule

2. *"I am going to stop trying to please you and I am going to stop pushing myself so hard"*

Rules Are Not Truths

After you have said your phrase, preferably out loud be aware of how much you believe the statement on a scale of 1-100 with 100 being total belief. Don't be surprised if your score is quite low. You are trying to change a thought habit of a lifetime!

Jessica says she finds it hard to express her anger to her father as she pictures him being dismissive towards her. She believes the positive statement 40% as its hard to imagine changing.

Now consider why you might not start to fully believe and live your statement. Who's life is it? Why should you not chose to start living your life in a way that is actually more reasonable and comfortable for you. Why are you giving so much power to the person who gave you the rule? How come their take on the world is better than yours? Be aware of the reaction you imagine they have to your statement – they may be dismissive, upset, angry, hurt. Part of regaining your power is stopping protecting your parents from the authentic you. As stated before disagreeing with part of what they taught you does not mean you do not love them

Jessica acknowledges that she has always given father a lot of power in her life. She starts to see that her own point of view is valid and that she cannot continue to lead her life in a way that suits him and yet causes her so many problems.

As a parent I cannot expect you as my child to be a clone of me. I need to respect that you are uniquely your own person even if that means that you think, feel or live your life very differently from me. Failure to do this means I fail as a parent. This clearly involves pain for the parent with the expectations and hopes that they may have had AND this is part of the challenge and pain of being a parent.

Old Rule-New Rule Checklist

If you want to change the mental blueprint of the rules you were given as a child you have to:

- Identify the rule and the emotion with which it was delivered
- Identify the emotion you feel about the rule
- Decide you no longer wish to accept and live by this rule
- Give the emotion back to the rule maker with a clear short statement which is preferably spoken out loud as if to them or is written down.
- Create a positive statement (a new rule) regarding the old rule
- Check how much you believe the statement 1 -100
- Debate with yourself why you cannot fully believe the statement
- Repeat the statement many times as you start to internalise the new rule
-

Actual Parent vs Internalised Historic Parent

Many clients struggle with standing up to their parents. To clarify, when I say parents I mean the internalised parent ie the image we have inside us of our parents. Sometimes we may need to stand up to a living breathing parent but very often what needs to change is the view we carry around of our parents in our head.

Internalised Historic Parent ...vs ...Actual Parent

Also, it is important to note that the Internalised Historic Parent may not be the same or hold the same views as the contemporary Actual Parent. Our view of our parent is often based on their behaviours when we were children. So, the bullying nagging mother from when we were five may still be in our mind as the Internalised Historic Parent whereas the Actual Parent twenty years on may have mellowed into someone who loves and supports us.

By the time Jessica had become an experienced nurse her father was treating her much more affectionately and listened to her point of view. However, Jessica held the Internalised Historic Parent as the bully he had been years before. She therefore often mis-read or misinterpreted what he said as she continually expected criticism. In the same way she heard her boss being demanding whereas it was Jessica who turned a request into a demand and became her own worst bully!"

Although your parent currently treats you well you may still need to address issues with the historic parent who you have internalised. If your parent still treats you badly and abusively then even more reason to deal with the Internalised Parent.

If you have become used to being abused, ignored, bullied, teased or dominated by members of your family you may well internalise this behaviour and practise it on yourself via your own Internal Critic. Clients often do not realise how harshly they treat themselves and it is only when you dig into their history you discover a bullying, critical mother or father whose attributes they have taken on:

"But that's not harsh, that's what I'm used to"

How You May Stop Yourself Re-making the Rules

Rejecting the old set of rules and creating new rules by which you live is a very powerful tool for regaining control and a sense of power and agency in your life. Being able to state how you felt/feel about the old rule and clearly express the new rule is crucial to your moving forward. Indeed, my experience would suggest you will remain trapped in the old patterns until such time as you can. However, there are a number of processes which may make it difficult for you to do this.

Approval

Most people enjoy the warm glow of approval from other people, especially their parents and siblings. As children we might paint a picture, dance a little dance or play a tune and our parents tell us we are wonderful (or not!). This can then become a tool by which parents exert control:

"If you do what I want then I will approve of you and give you love"

We can become used to this approval and then after a while it feels difficult to do things where there is no approval or that worse, we enter into conflict with our parents. Love becomes conditional. Alternatively our parents might be very dominant and it feels frightening to contradict their wishes. The need for approval can become part of a wider process which is called confluence. We will discuss this shortly.

Exercise 2.5: Approval

Reflect on the degree to which you needed your parents approval. Write down particular ways in which you needed their approval. Consider the degree to which you currently need approval from your family, friends or colleagues. Be careful if you strongly feel you do not need their approval as this may be a form of denial ie because you did not get their approval you say " Ok well I do not need your approval anyway". Holding this sort of anger is not a resolution but rather a temporary way of dealing with such difficulty.

Globalising vs Discriminating

Clients often find it difficult to reject anything they were taught as children as this feels a betrayal of their parents. Realising that we can love someone AND dislike certain behaviours or attitudes they hold is often the best way to resolve this. Rejecting one or two things does not mean you totally reject them. If you parents had very black and white thinking it may "feel" as though you are rejecting all of them ie "You are either for me or against me!" Actually you are using an adult faculty which is you are choosing to discriminate. You are saying "This piece of what you taught me was useful and this piece was not and that is fine".

Idealised Fantasy vs Reality

We often hold a picture somewhere in our minds of The Perfect Family populated with a perfect Mum and Dad and brothers and sisters; a sort of virtual family. Sadly, for most of us our families are not perfect they are a mixture of awful, wonderful, average, great etc. What is crucial is that we do not hold onto some perfect picture and then spend our lives yearning for something different. Generally speaking people do not change very much so if your father has historically not been very demonstrative and does not easily express his feelings the chances are he will continue like that. If as a son I dream of having a father who I can sit down and have a long heart-to-heart with I am probably destined to a life of frustration.

Key Idea:

I have to work with what is. Not what I wish

How I Learnt to Merge with Others and Avoid Conflict

The following is a classic psychological pattern in the emotional blueprint of someone who over-eats. Understanding and changing this pattern can rapidly enable you to assert a stronger sense of who you are. This in turn will lead to you feeling emotionally clearer and more in control. When you feel like this you will have no need to over-eat.

In typical development the mother's and baby's needs are so intertwined that there is a special close bond. As the child's identity develops so there is often more conflict. As the child grows so she increasingly asserts her needs and her difference. By teenagehood there may be a breakdown in the relationship as the sense of difference becomes more profound. Usually by late teens to mid twenties there is a sense of mutal respect. Child and parent may have different ideas and views but they nonetheless can love and respect one another.

Rules Are Not Truths

Where the parent is very dominant and/or insecure this process breaks down. The young child may go to assert their difference by, for example, choosing to wear a particular article of clothing. The parent dis-approves and effectively says:

"If you chose to be different I will stop approving of and loving you"

The child is faced with an impossible dilemma. They want to be loved but they deeply need to be themselves. Children will often accede to what their parents wish but then give up on their own sense of uniqueness and individuality. This sense of identity merger is called confluence. Difference is subjugated in favour of "harmony". Conflict is avoided because the emotional price is somehow too high. The child is now in what is called a merged or confluent relationship.

This pattern then gets played out in adult life by the individual finding it hard both to say "no" and to define boundaries. They live with a sense that they should always please their boss, colleagues, friends and relations. As in their childhood the price for this "equanimity" is high; an underlying resentment and anger that somehow they do not get what they need and eventually of course a high toll upon their physical and emotional well-being.

Painfully, confluent individuals have to re-define the balance between their own needs and that of the world. This requires a difficult re-calibration of what is "selfish" and what is actually healthy and wise:

"How can I stop for lunch when I have such a big case-load!"

"I can't just say to my manager that I won't take on another project because I'm maxed up".

"What will my colleagues say if I say no".

Rocking the boat is a long way out of the confluent individual's comfort zone so it is often easier to just remain stressed – until of course they become physically ill and have to take a long hard look at that thirty year pattern!

Exercises 2.6: Identity Merger

How would you rate your degree of identity merger with one or both parents.

On a scale of 1 -100 how merged would you consider yourself to have been?

How merged are you currently with people close to you?

Did you go through a period when you rebelled against the identity merger. If so, how successful was this rebellion? Did you fully break away and create your own identity. Does it still matter to you what your parents think?

Can you hear their point of view and still come to your own conclusion?

Confluence, Approval & The Lock-In

Working with clients who over-eat I am struck by how many are moderately to highly identity merged. The greater the merger the greater the sense of difficulty with standing up to the Internalised Historic Parent and the greater the difficulty of course in dealing with their own Internal Critic.

What causes this difficulty? The difficulty arises because there is a dual mechanism operating with these internalised rules. For example:

As a child Jessica's father told her that she should do as she was told. On numerous occasions when she purposefully or accidentally disobeyed him he became so angry that she would shake with fear. Soon he only had to look at her a certain way and she would feel the fear. She learnt that it was easier and that she felt safer to do what he said. Over time she did not really notice his anger so much but just became used to doing what he wished.

So, Jessica learnt three things:

"I must do what I am told by people in authority"

"If I do not something very unpleasant will happen"

"This is normal and anyway, whatever, I should protect my parents".

The "something unpleasant" was her sense of fear and the feeling of that in her body which again become automatic to the extent that her father did not even need to shout. The Lock-In is the sense that something, however abusive or even minor, becomes normal and most importantly we should protect our parents from emotional pain. If we think of this as a process, it might look a bit like this:

- Parent "You will accord with my wishes if not I will withdraw my love"

- Child " OK, I'll give up my sense of being myself but I need you to love me".

- Parent: OK, but if you get that wrong I'll be furious or tell you you are killing me. You should agree with me and take care of me"
- Child" OK, whatever I just want to forget all this stuff and act like it's normal... and actually I just want to protect you"

The child is therefore emotionally blackmailed by the parent's anger or vulnerability into giving up on their own sense of identity. Fast forward to the child being an adult and we will have someone who is very vulnerable to overeating because they cannot face expressing themselves or deal with conflict.

Exercise 2.7: Challenging the Lock-In

Start to run through the Old Rule-New Rule checklist below. You may find this exercise difficult. I will break each stage down to help support you. Be aware how and when you start to find the exercise difficult. Notice if your body tightens up as you think about the exercise. What feelings do you have towards your parents or towards yourself as you do this? Take each stage slowly and reflect on it before you move on to the next stage. You cannot rush this!

- Identify the old rule and the emotion(s) with which it was delivered
- Identify the emotion you feel about the rule
- Decide you no longer wish to accept and live by this rule

- Give the emotion back to the rule-maker with a clear short statement which is preferably spoken out loud as if to them or is written down.

- Create a positive statement (a new rule) regarding the old rule

- Check how much you believe the statement 1 -100

- Debate with yourself why you cannot fully believe the statement

- Repeat the statement many times as you start to internalise the new rule

Example:

- *Jessica identifies that she should always had to do what her father wished. This was delivered with a mixture of anger and insecurity ie if she was different he would not be able to control her.*
- *She feels hurt, angry and sad that he wanted to control her*
- *She decides she no longer wishes to accept this control from him*
- *She creates a short statement:*
- *"I am no longer willing to be controlled by you or (linking it to her present life) anyone else".*
- *She create a positive statement:*

"I will live my own life and be my own person with my differences. I will expect to be treated with respect"

- *She rates her belief in this statement: Initially 75% of her believes it.*
- *When she debates why these statements shouldn't be true she starts to believe them further*
- *With repetition she starts to more fully believe her statements*

Clients often find it hard to complete or even begin this exercise. Typical responses to the request to do this exercise are:

I can't remember any rules".	We all learn rules they are there somewhere!
"I feel bad talking negatively about my parents.	You can love them and still disagree with elements of what they taught.
"This feels like I'm letting them down"	And maybe if you don't deal with this you let yourself down
"What they did was normal"	Normal for your family, not necessarily healthy.
"They'll get upset/angry"	These are all forms of emotional blackmail which eventually you have to, safely, face
"They'll say I'm killing them"	
"They'll get violent, it's too dangerous. I don't feel safe"	

Rules Are Not Truths

Breaking free from this sort of identity merged emotional blackmail takes courage and energy. As a 50 year old client with a "successful life" said to me today:

"But if I don't go on fulfilling my father's (and every other man's) expectations who will I be"

It's scary to be different. It's scary to invite your parent's disapproval – even if that is your Internalised Parent. Yet the question remains: who will you be if you do not stand-up to these demands? Your parents created the emotional blueprint for all your future contact with other people . If you do not confront their demands you will simply re-cycle the old patterns of suppressing your emotions, disconnecting from your body and not expressing your needs. When you do this you are likely to over-eat. In the end you sometimes have to take a deep breath and dive off the board in the belief that you can and will survive. Let's consider that list of reasons why clients say that they cannot make a clear statement to the their parent(s) rejecting the old rule:

   1. " I can't remember any rules"   Try this:

Exercise 2.8: Shoulds

Write down a list of all the things you believe you should or should not do. Check your list and consider how many of these "should" were learnt from your parents. These are your old rules. Now try the main exercise above.

   2. "I feel bad talking negatively about my parents"

It is quite possible to love someone and to dislike an element of their behaviour or a particular aspect of them or what they taught you. Part of confluent thinking is it is very black and white "You either love me or hate me". Can you allow your relationship with your parents to become more sophisticated ie to dislike elements of their behaviour but to still love them.

3." Talking about my parents feels like I'm letting them down"

In exploring yourself this is not about creating blame rather it is you trying to understand the software which makes you tick. Your parents did the best they could for you and we can only parent well to the degree that we were well parented. Where we have learnt poor patterns or rules we have to find new ways to re-parent ourselves (more on this later). The only way we can do this is to examine our history and how our parents behaved.

4. "What my parents taught was normal"

Well it was normal for your family but was that helpful or healthy for you? If you live comfortably with rules you were given by your parents that is fine. However, if you find yourself unhappy or in conflict with them it is maybe time to examine them and yourself more deeply.

5. "My parents will get angry"

6.. "They'll get upset, they'll get sad, they'll say I'm killing them" "They'll get violent, it's too dangerous –I don't feel safe"

As children, adult's emotions especially of anger and upset can seem very big and scary. Sometimes it is appropriate they are upset if we placed ourselves in danger or were disobedient. However, if they became emotional because they were demanding some sort of confluent behaviour on your part as a child then this is clearly emotionally manipulative.

Some clients who find it difficult to confront the Internalised Parent do so because of their fear of some kind of emotional or aggressive retribution. It reminds me of Oliver in Oliver Twist saying "Please Sir, can I have some more!" Faced with thinking or visualising their parent clients can regress and become the small child victim who could be beaten or abused. In a therapy setting I might sit alongside a client who has become small and frightened and support them to begin to find a voice and to speak up for themselves.

Exercise 2.9: Standing up to an Aggressive Internalised Parent

Depending on the level of aggression you experienced as a child this may seem an exercise which is on a range from difficult to …….impossible. Being able to achieve this exercise as with any requires that you may need to do it in small enough steps and with sufficient support to feel "safe enough". Indeed, feeling sufficiently safe whilst stepping a little out of your comfort zone is the key to achieving any change. Try to be compassionate with yourself in achieving this exercise.

If you experienced high levels of aggression or violence you may want to imagine some way of containing your parent before you speak to them. This might include speaking to them through a reinforced screen which they cannot get through. One client I worked with imagined placing their parent in a secure cage which was impossible for them to break out of. What is important is that you feel safe enough as you try to speak with them.

Another way to support yourself with this exercise is to either imagine a trusted friend or relation sitting with you or actually inviting someone you really trust to be with you as attempt the exercise.

1. Firstly picture your parent you wish to speak with. You may picture them physically contained or constrained or not depending on your level of fear.

2. Be aware of your own reaction as you picture them. If you start to feel anxious breathe deeply from your abdomen. (See p. 52) Try to ground yourself.

3. Make a statement which rejects their treatment of you:

    "I am no longer prepared to be bullied and intimidated by you"

4. Be aware of their reaction – dismissive, aggressive, indifferent

5. Allow yourself to hold on to your own value and opinion. Make statement which affirms this

"It's fine for me to be different to you, even if you strongly disagree"

6. Again be aware of their reaction and yours. Make sure you keep breathing fully

7. Integration: If you manage to achieve this, fine now over the coming weeks and months be aware of where in your current life you allow yourself to be intimidated or bullied. Ensuring you breathe fully repeat the statements in the exercise until you start to completely believe them. This may take some time to reach complete belief but hey you are trying to change the habit of a lifetime! The next stage as your confidence grows to actually stand-up to the person currently bullying or intimidating you and make the statements or some form of them directly to them.

If you could not complete the exercise you may need to consider ways to imagine containing your parent further or create more support such as having another person present with you. If this is too difficult you may want to think about getting professional help to enable you to manage the feelings the exercise may evoke. If this is the case again be compassionate with yourself around your needs and look to what can best support you.

To take this exercise to the next level you could imagine your parent actually in the room with you but still contained or constrained if required. This will give the exercise more immediacy and emotional impact so you need to ensure you feel sufficiently supported and protected.

Although this exercise can be very difficult I would encourage you to try it as I have seen many clients start to turn their lives around from the point of daring to complete this exercise

Jessica became tearful when I suggested this exercise. She said that when she really thought about it she found her father's anger as a child very frightening. We agreed we needed to make it safer so she imagined him inside a cage made of steel and manacled to a chair. As we reached the point of her trying to say the statement she became visibly frightened. I encourage her to breathe deeply and for the duration of the exercise she asked me to place my hand in the small of her back to feel some support. She made the statement: "I am no longer willing to be bullied and intimidated by you". She checked her reaction – she felt wobbly and imagined his reaction would be dismissive and scornful. She made the second statement. " Its fine for me to be different from you even if you strongly disagree". She imagined he became very angry and abusive and told her she was nothing.

Then a smile broke out on her face and she said. "You know I'm suddenly not so afraid. He's sort of pathetic. He needs me to be like him because he's too frightened to allow me to be my own person. He fears he wont be able to control me any more. I won't be his "little girl". "Well I'm not a little girl any more I'm my own person and if you do not like that its sad but you are not going to stop me being who I am. I don't need your approval any more."

Jessica broke through the hypnotism of the Lock-In ie that the rule is the truth and finally realised she did not need to accord with what her father wanted or even that she need be afraid of him

Rules Are Not Truths

Exercise 2.10: Standing up to an Emotionally Manipulative Internalised Parent

This exercise is similar to the last one without the need for visualising any sort of constraint because the danger from them is more focussed on emotional abuse. This might include parents who demand a confluent relationship or in some way did not allow you to develop in your own unique and special way.

1. Firstly picture your parent you wish to speak with or picture them sitting opposite you

2. Be aware of your own reaction as you picture them. If you start to feel anxious breathe deeply from your abdomen. (See p. 52) Try to ground yourself.

3. Make a statement which rejects their expectations of you:

    "I was not brought into this world to fulfil your expectations"

4. Be aware of their reaction – dismissive, aggressive, indifferent

5. Allow yourself to hold on to your own value and opinion

6. Make statement which affirms this

7. "It's fine for me to be different from you, even if you strongly disagree. I do not need your approval to be ok"

8. Again be aware of their reaction and yours. Make sure you keep breathing fully

Many clients who have had emotionally manipulative parents will say:

"But I should fulfil their expectations!"When they say this I often counter with:"I'm a fifty four year old man ...should I live my life according to my mother's expectations?"And they all say "Yes, of course" ... no I'm joking, they say "Of course, not". And the counter to that is "So why should you live your life according to your parents expectations?" And then they often look quite blank and say "I don't know, I just should".

So, we are back to what I called the Lock-In ie that I learn a rule "I should meet your expectations" and then magically, hypnotically I forget this is a rule which can be changed and then I take it as the truth.

Key Idea: Rules we are given as children are not THE TRUTH – they are a human construction which we can agree with, dispute or change. They may be useful to our current life or not – we need to decide what works for us currently

Being Equal

Below the sense of being merged with my parents or with other people is often the feeling that I am not equal with them. I have learnt to be subordinate or somehow smaller than them. This sense of inferiority can again cause us to suppress our true feelings or reactions to others. This again, in turn, can frequently lead to over-eating.

Underlying dealing with difficult Internalised Parents is often our sense of equality or rather the lack of it. As children there is an in-built power imbalance. Learning to develop a sense of equality with our parents can be difficult. Especially with strong cultural rules, such as "You should respect your parents". Well I agree I want to be respectful to my parents AND that respect should be a two way street.

Part of bringing a child into the world is to allow them to become the unique and special person they are irrespective of my dreams or expectations as a parent. So, I would want to respect and consider seriously what my parents said and ultimately it is my life and I need to decide what is wise for me even if that means I fall flat on my face. It may be painful but it is the only way to really learn anything! As parents we need to love enough to be able to stand back and let our children make the mistakes they need to make.

Exercise 2.11 " I am Your Equal"

Try saying the sentence below in your mind whilst picturing a variety of people. Note your reaction and then consider on a scale 1 -100 how much you believe the sentence to be true.

Imagine saying to your boss "I am your equal"

Imagine saying to your partner "I am your equal"

Imagine saying to your colleague "I am your equal"

Imagine saying to your mother "I am your equal"

Imagine saying to your father "I am your equal"

If you do not feel equal with all these people consider in what way you are not equal. Some may have a role or skill set you feel is superior. Well, we all have skills or are developing some. I know something about psychotherapy – does that make me superior to you? You may know a lot about teaching or being a mother or hang gliding does it make you superior to me? If we put our skill sets to one side how is this person actually better than you? Today I'm your therapist tomorrow you're a para-medic saving my life! Roles may give power but roles can change so does that make people superior to you? When we get down to our humanness it seems to me we are equal. Believing or certainly starting to believe in your equality with all will allow you to feel freer to express yourself and especially not to be abused.

Integration:

To integrate this exercise try saying, to yourself, "I'm your equal" to everyone you meet. Notice who you do or do not feel equal with? Also, be aware when you feel superior!? I would suggest that this is equally unhealthy as feeling inferior. Indeed, you might see superiority as another form of inferiority – if I am truly secure about my achievements why would I need to feel superior!! An attitude of superiority can lead to you communicating a sense of contempt for others and if the feeling is there, even subtly, people will pick it up and react accordingly. This can be very damaging to any relationship. Try to cultivate operating from a place where you simply are equal, this will enable you to feel good about yourself and to treat people well.

Conflict-Avoidance

Another strand which runs through the inability to stand up to those who gave us inadequate or inappropriate rules is the avoidance of conflict. As children the anger of adults or simply their disapproval can be something very frightening. We may feel physically afraid or that in some way will be humiliated or shamed if we enter into conflict. Adults are so much more powerful than children.

If we have become used to a confluent relationship we may well at some stage in our life come to the following sort of conclusions:

"Anything for a quiet life"

"I can't stand rowing"

"I heard enough shouting as a child, I don't need anymore"

"If I get into an argument there's no accounting for what I may do. My anger scares me"

"I know I should stand up for myself but I don't want to hurt anyone"

These are all different examples of conflict-avoidance. In their own way they are all valid I can see the logic of them. Yet if we are trying to establish the most essential rules by which we are going to live for the rest of our lives it maybe that we need to be prepared to stand-up for what we believe in. This will involve a degree of conflict, a degree of discomfort yet the prize will be starting to experience a far greater degree of freedom within yourself!

Clients who find conflict difficult often do so because they lack the skills of assertion. They either tend to collapse in the face of conflict or they become enraged and scare themselves. Assertion requires you learn the middle way.

Exercise 2.12: The Yes-No Game

I use the following exercise a lot with clients who find assertion difficult. You need to find a friend to do this one with . It's fun and it's also very revealing so make sure you choose a good friend! The first part is an analysis of the problem of assertion. Try doing this before you read the section called Review.

Firstly, imagine a typical scenario of conflict at home or work.

Yes-No Scenario

Person A (Your friend, in their role as your boss, your partner etc) is going to say one word only which is "Yes". This word represents their desire for you to take a particular course of action which you do NOT wish to do. For example we imagine Person A is asking Person B to do work an extra shift etc

Person B (which will be you) will say one word only which is "No"

Person A needs to try saying "Yes" in a variety of ways: Quietly, forcefully, wheedling, jokey but always just the one word. Imagine you are trying to batter or cajole the other person into submission but if they become emotional ie tearful or angry then quickly conclude the session. Try to be observant about how Person B says No!.

Person B simply say "No" however comes naturally to you. At the same time be aware of how you feel emotionally and physically as Person A keeps addressing you.

Review

Person B feeds back how they felt doing this exercise. Did they feel strong or weak? Did any voice tone from Person A undermine them more than another? Did they feel anything physically? How did they feel emotionally? How would they score themselves on their ability to be assertive given that

Rules Are Not Truths

experience 1- 10 – 10 being very assertive.

Person A feeds back what they noticed. This can include things like:

Voice quality

Eye contact

Belief in saying "No"

Smiling

Pace

Breathing

Coaching

When I coach clients on assertion they will usually have just done the Yes-No game so I will feed back on the categories above. I might use the following type of statements.

You didn't sound like you believed your "No"

You were barely breathing

You kept smiling at me

You found it hard to give me eye contact

Your voice was very quiet, hard, angry

You responded at my pace

Self Belief: In order to be assertive we need to believe that it is ok for us to have a particular point of view and express it. So, maybe it is time for you to start to believe it is absolutely fine for you to have a point of view and to express it clearly and unequivocally.

Breathing: To be assertive we need to breathe deeply and slowly. In any conflict situation it helps if you get your own physiology under control as best you can. So, practise breathing away from the conflict zone.

Smiling: Smiling whilst you say "No" or refuse something sends a massive double message. Given that most of us read body language in a micro second and according to research believe body language far more than words what you are really saying when you smile and say "No" are three things:

1. You are really saying "Yes"
2. You want me to approve of you
3. And you may also trying to protect me from the pain of your saying "No"

Smiling whilst saying "No" sends a huge double message that you are uncertain or ambiguous about saying it. If you say "No" and I disapprove of this you have to learn to accept it. No means no, and sometimes people do not like to hear it. However, we all need at times to refuse to do things to support ourselves physically or emotionally.

Rules Are Not Truths

When clients find it difficult to say "No" I will suggest they imagine we are good colleagues and I say "No" to them regarding some particular issue. Their response is invariably "Oh, that's fine". So, it seems it is ok for other people to say "No" but not for you? Again, they often look blank and nonplussed. It is clear to them that logically it should be ok for them to say "No" but somehow they have been programmed to believe that it is not ok. Returning to the first point we have to develop the self belief that this is my life, my body, my time, my energy and it is entirely reasonable if I say "No". Clearly if I always said no this might well become an issue. If I am generally in good and collegial relations with people then to sometimes say "No" is reasonable and will usually be accepted as such. If it is not then clearly some sort of discussion is required with that person.

Eye Contact: Eye contact is a hugely important part of human communication. Being able to hold eye contact suggests a certain degree of confidence in itself. You are communicating your sense of equality and the fact that you see the other person clearly. Dropping eye contact whilst saying "No" suggests a sort of ambiguity and lack of confidence or an implied submission. Turning it into a staring contest however suggests aggression and moves you off the fulcrum of being assertive.

Voice Quality: Doing this exercise clients can either speak very quietly or inappropriately loudly. Your voice tone again communicates a lot about how you feel about saying "No". Speaking quietly can also communicate an ambiguity about your confidence in this matter. Speaking loudly suggests an aggression which can also be experienced as a lack of confidence

Pace: If you simply respond in a mechanical way each time I say "Yes" it sounds as though I'm dictating the pace. Respond in your own time.

Repeat the Yes-No Game

Repeat the exercise but this time:

- Remember to believe in your right to say "No"
- Use slow deep breathing to support yourself
- Do not smile. Let your face be neutral
- With feedback from your partner first, raise your voice if you were speaking quietly. Maintain your level and an even tone but do not shout.
- Go at your pace. Try pausing and breathing before you respond

Exercise 2.13: Homework

Having explored how to say "No" in the exercise now try this in your life. Firstly become aware of the times when you would like to say "No" . Become aware of how often you want to say "No" but do not. Choose an issue, probably something small initially where you disagree or want to do something differently and try actually saying "No". Bear in mind all the points in the exercise. Notice how successful or not you were with this and review it using the checklists above

Closure

Feelings and the sensations which accompany them have their own life. For example if I say something and you feel hurt this emotion will continue to resonate within you until you have found a way to close the emotion. Individuals who are disconnected from their physical/emotional process will have lots of un-concluded emotional reactions operating within them. If they also operate according to rules which do not allow them to discuss or express their emotions these feelings will be held within them often without much awareness.

As we become more aware of our sensory-emotional life so we will find that we have to start finding ways to bring about emotional closure.

Having become aware of her anxiety and anger with her boss Jessica needs to find some degree of closure. She therefore might:

Write her feelings in a diary

- Talk to a friend

- Write a letter to her boss about the issues which she does not send. Write the letter to her boss and send it

- Talk to a therapist and rehearse how she might talk to her boss

- Talk directly with her boss about her concerns

- In addition she might write down and or talk to others about her anger with herself. With support she might consider treating herself with greater compassion and to stop recycling her father's critical voice.

Exercise.2.14: Closure

Repeat the Body Zones exercise in Chapter One, track through the 10 zones of your body checking what sensations you discover and what images or emotions you associate with this sensation. Having completed this exercise now consider the sensations and emotions you discovered. Ask yourself the simple question: What sort of closure does this emotion require?

- Can I initially write down how I feel?

- Do I need to talk to a friend? Imagine what you might say.

- Do I need to write a letter I do not send or one that I do? Try writing a letter you do not send. Read it out to yourself or a friend that you trust.

- Do I need to talk directly with the person or people who are causing me distress? Imagine what you might say to them.

- Is all of this too much and do I need to talk to a counsellor? Try some of the above before you pick up the phone – you might be surprised what you can achieve by externalising the feeling ie writing or talking.

Work through the different emotions you discovered and see if you can take one or more actions towards resolving the feelings. Much distress is caused by our inability to provide closure on our emotions. Emotions which remain un-closed continue to repeat like a tape loop going round and round until we have found a way to resolve them. With the right resolution the feeling rapidly departs and we recover our equilibrium. So, in my early example of saying something which hurts you, if I later clearly empathise with your upset and say a genuine apology the chances are we both move on and the feeling of discomfort you experienced will recede.

Key Ideas: 4: Unresolved emotions will continue to function inside you until you resolve them. Commit to resolving these emotions through some of the suggested routes described above

Over-Eating: A Psychological Profile

Below is a summary checklist of some of the psychological qualities of someone over-eats. How many are true of you:

Puts everyone else's needs first

Cannot connect with their own sensations/feelings very easily

Cannot easily express emotions

Certainly cannot meet the needs which arise out of these feelings

Cannot maintain boundaries

Difficulty with assertion. Cannot say "No"

Feels stressed and demanded of by their friends, work and family

Being approved of is very important. Seek approval from parents and others.

Often a bad life/work balance

Dislikes conflict

Summary

- In the preceding section we have explored the importance of the rules we learnt as children. We've seen how rules can become internalised to the degree that we forget that the rule is a creation and the rule then becomes a truth or a fact. Clearly, some rules we learnt are very helpful, such as "Do not walk into a busy road" others, such as " Don't rock the boat!" may be helpful at times but not if you apply them to all situations.

- We have learnt that most of us have a whole heap of rules around issues such as our body, food and most importantly ourselves. We've learnt where we fit in terms of family position and how this may affect us

- We've learnt how to distinguish a useful rule from a not so useful rule. Does it enhance your life. How to support ourselves to stand up to our parents re. Bad Rules and how to create a New Guideline!!

- We learnt about the crucial difference between an Actual Parent and an Internalised Historic Parent and we've learnt how to stand-up to an aggressive and or manipulative parent

- We've learnt about the idea of Confluence and associated ideas of equality, approval and the notion of The Lock-In

Rules Are Not Truths

which helps us forget that rules are created by human beings and that rules are not Truths or facts.

- We considered the importance of conflict avoidance and the development of assertion through the Yes-No Game

- We considered the importance of closure in relation to outstanding feelings.

CHAPTER 3

How We Learn to Bury our Feelings

In her wonderful book *Why Love Matters* Sue Gerhardt describes how it is love and affection which helps to form the brain of the developing baby. The sensation of holding, the intimate gaze of the mother, the caresses and stroking all help to stimulate the release of various neuro-transmitting chemicals. The chemicals generate both pleasure but also help the brain to build a stable sense of the child existing in a secure environment.

It has been shown that babies deprived of this love and security have a less developed pre-frontal cortex and anterior cingulate – areas concerned with social interaction. Further research has shown that this early lack of development affects them developing lasting intimate relationships.

Whilst love affects the early development of the brain current research strongly indicates that the brain exhibits plasticity, that is, it is capable of on-going organic change and development. This quality accounts for why counselling and psychotherapy can be so effective as the therapist is helping the client to re-structure not only their thoughts and feelings but the brain itself.

How We Learn To Bury Our Feelings

Repeated inputs from parents will create neural circuits in the brain. These neural networks repeated over time become "just the way it is" – a bit like sheep creating a particular track over open downland, after a while they all go down the same path. "We've never been a family to socialise –we just like to be together". Therapy can help to explore the current path and maybe look at alternative paths. As the client is angry about or grieves for the old path so they start to open the space to allow the creation of a new way forward. This new way is based upon what they need rather than what they "should" do.

So, clearly love matters at a biological as well as psychological level. Louis Cozolino has described how heroin helps to release some of the same chemicals as those released when we feel loved. He suggests that, in a sense addicts are looking to reproduce the sensation of feeling loved through taking the drug. Chocolate similarly helps in the release of chemicals which mimic in part the sense of being loved. Which would account for the research that given the choice between sex and chocolate most women will go for the chocolate!! What they would do if the choice is between a man with, what one of my clients calls, Advanced Listening Skills and chocolate is unknown, although my bet would still be on the chocolate!!

Family Rules About Emotions

In the last chapter we were exploring the rules we live by– the habitual paths we, like the sheep, automatically go down and becoming more conscious about whether these rules are supportive or not. Some rules just apply to specific situations others are what I call Meta-Rules ie they apply to the very way we function. They are a default position.

How We Learn To Bury Our Feelings

One particular set of Meta-Rules are the **rules about emotionsthemselves**. To investigate this consider the following questions

Exercise 3.1: Family Rules about Emotions

- To what extent was it ok for you to **express** your feelings in your childhood family?

- Were feelings **discussed** as a part of family life?

- Were your feelings,"**taken into consideration**" when decisions were made about your life?

- Were you encouraged to **explore or reflect upon** your emotions?

- What did your parents **model** to you about emotions and feelings?

- Was there a difference in attitude about emotions between your parents?

- Write a brief sketch of your parents describing their different temperaments. When you have written the sketch consider what elements of their temperament you have either taken on or reacted against and created some other particular approach to your emotions ie if your mother was very volatile you may have decided to contain your own emotions quite strongly. Be aware therefore of the effect their emotional patterns had upon you.

How We Learn To Bury Our Feelings

Notice the highlighted words above used in reference to emotions and feelings: expressed, discussed, explore, reflect upon, model. Consider the degree to which you do express, discuss, reflect upon etc your feelings **currently** OR whether you close down and suppress your emotional life. Having reflected upon the emotional tone or atmosphere of your childhood you may be aware of various things:

Look at the table and consider which description is most like your own family:

There was a lot of emotion expressed	There was little emotion expressed
There was space to reflect upon emotions	Emotions were never reflected upon
My personal feelings were considered	My personal feelings were not considered
My parents owned and acknowledged their own feelings	My parents did not own their feelings
It was ok to be "different"	It was not ok to be different. I had to conform to the values and ideas of my parents

What all of this will hopefully start to reveal to you is how emotionally intelligent or articulate your family were. Do not be surprised if they were not especially aware! Of course even with parents who are reasonably emotionally intelligent it is very easy within the pressure cooker of the family for difficulties to develop.

How We Learn To Bury Our Feelings

Exercise 3.2: The Main Family Rules about Emotions

From the exercises above I would encourage you to consider what the top 3 or 4 rules were in your family regarding emotion. Whether these rules you experienced were implied, modelled or overt write them down.

To return to our old friend Jessica, if she considered this question the answers would be:

" My Mum was not that interested in my feelings and my Dad insisted I see things his way so the main rule I learnt was:

"Your feelings are not important"

My Mum always sided with my Dad and put him first" so I guess I also learnt:

"Other people's feeling come first, especially men's"

When I occasionally really did fight back and try to stand up for myself the feedback was:

"Don't you start getting above yourself ie putting your feelings first " and

"Whatever you do you won't be successful... because our feelings are more important than yours!.

Working over the years with many clients who have had over-eating as a primary or secondary problem it is apparent that they were nearly all clients who had learnt to suppress their feelings.

These clients main model for dealing with other people's behaviour and emotions was as shown in the diagram on page 50.

How We Learn To Bury Our Feelings

Something would occur which would cause an emotional reaction. Based on the old rules about emotions they would suppress their reaction. This in turn would lead to a state of emotional numbness where nothing particular was felt. This would create a state of disconnection between the mind/emotions/feeling/thoughts and the body. What was left was a sense of something missing; an empty feeling. This emptiness is either interpreted as "hunger" or just a generalised sense of "needing something". What often fills this vacuum is food - see diagram over-leaf.

With a big disconnect going on between mind and body there is a sense of being on automatic as they reach out to the fridge or the biscuit tin. Whilst this brings a temporary relief it may often require repeated eating to really meet the sense of emptiness. Of course this brief period of release is usually soon followed by a sense of guilt, shame or disgust that "again" you have let yourself down. You did not have the "willpower" to resist, you feel unhappy with your lack of resolve and even unhappier with the feelings of bloatedness and the loss of power over controlling you weight. As the food is digested this acute feeling of self-hatred will often resolve but what is left is a generalised sense of depression that your life is not within your control and somehow you are weak. Life starts again but of course whilst you suppress your emotional reactions and the meeting of your most essential needs the chances are you will repeat this cycle the next time something difficult or challenging occurs again.

Explore the diagram and see if this applies to you. We are all unique and your personal model may be somewhat different but it will probably include all or some of the stages outlined. Notice how Stage.2 is such a crucial point as the old rule kicks in and you start to behave in a semi-automatic way. This is such an important point at which change can occur if you are able to challenge the old rules.

How We Learn To Bury Our Feelings

Suppressing Emotion With Food in 8 Stages

1. Emotional Reaction: Someone says or does something to which you have an emotional reaction

2. You **Suppress Emotion** based on old parental rule

"It's not ok to have or express feelings" OR

Rule: "Other people come first" etc

8. Get back on with life, push away feeling negative, depressed & powerless

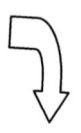

3. Feel Numb/Disconnected

7. Self Criticise: "I'm weak, let myself down". Feel bloated, fat. "Need Something" sensation recurs ie need to feel stronger

4. "Need Something Sensation" Interpret this as need for food or taste of food

5. Over-Eat to avoid feelings

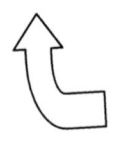

6. Temporary Relief from "Need Something". The sensation of food masks the emotion, temporarily.

How We Learn To Bury Our Feelings

Control Mechanisms re. Emotion

Consider your family rules relating to emotion. They usually contain elements of criticism: "Your ideas/behaviours/being is not ok" AND coercion: "Do as we do or there will be sanctions".

The control mechanisms related to the family rules on emotion usually involve all or some of the following:

You will be openly criticised: "Why are you getting so upset, grow up?"

You will be teased: "Oh is didums upset!"

You will be manipulated: "Don't tell me how your feeling, you're killing me!"

You will be shamed & humiliated : "Look at her, what an idiot, she's crying over nothing!".

You will be ignored: "What did you say?"

You will be threatened with physical abuse.: "I don't care how you feel, shut up or you'll get a slap"

In the same way that we can internalise the voice of our parents generally we tend to powerfully internalise the rules we learnt from them about emotions.

Exercise 3.3 Family Rules & Self Talk

Part.1

Consider how your family controlled the expression or consideration of emotion. Try to remember specific examples as detailed above and write them down.

How We Learn To Bury Our Feelings

Part.2

Consider your examples and reflect on whether your own "self talk" currently includes these sorts of ways of talking. Self talk includes ways we might encourage, reassure OR criticize ourselves ie we do something wrong and internally we attack ourselves "Oh there you go again, you idiot!".

Self Talk

Usually self talk is closely based upon what we learnt as children. We no longer therefore need our parents to criticize us as we have very efficiently internalised their voice. This is especially true in our attitudes towards our emotions. Cognitive behaviourists call self talk "automatic thoughts" ie little thoughts or comments which automatically kick in as a commentary on what we do. I was just watching a racing driver on the television cross the winning line. As he did so he cried "Yes, yes, yes, my beauty!!" For that moment as he apparently talked to his car, he was talking to and encouraging himself. He gave himself positive self talk which no doubt helped if he did this as he drove around the circuit.

Suppressing emotion does not get rid of the underlying feeling it simply manifests in a different way ie you may get a headache (headaches often relate to un-expressed anger in my experience) or some other physical symptom. Similarly, you may be irritable with the wrong people or as discussed end up over-eating.

How We Learn To Bury Our Feelings

Exercise 3.4: Letter to Your Parents

Take some time when you can be alone. Write a letter to your parents. **THIS IS A LETTER YOU ARE NOT GOING TO SEND.** The topic of the letter is going to be "What it was like being your daughter/son….". Detail the positives as you remember them and the negatives. Conclude with what you need to do to move on from the difficult parts of your childhood. In terms of attitudes to emotions try to state how you wish to deal with your own emotional life in future. ie

"It's fine for me to have emotions, to express them and to get support for myself in regard to my emotions. From now on I want to offer myself more compassion in terms of my feelings". Remember you can love people and still disagree with them.

Caring Cinderella

One particular personality trait that includes the extreme suppression or retroflection of feeling is what I call Caring Cinderella. This is mostly found in women for predominantly cultural reasons however there are no doubt some male Cinderellas around as well!! Whilst men suppress their emotions and over-eat because of this they do so for somewhat different reasons which I will detail shortly. Caring Cinderella is usually based upon 3 rules working together to create an especially focussed lack of compassion and care for oneself:

As a child the following rules are either taken on-board from the behaviour of the parents or arise as a reaction to their behaviour

How We Learn To Bury Our Feelings

- I should be there for everyone and support them"
- "I should show no needs of my own"
- "I should be perfect"

The Caring Cinderella is usually what I also call a conditioned carer in that they have often been raised with a strong imperative to rescue and take care of others. This may include caring for one or both parents or for other children in the family. Whilst this is clearly a humane thing to do when it becomes a default position ie "My role is to care for everyone!" then it can become problematic. In my work with healthcare workers they often arrive at my door because of their inability to self-care. When challenged on this it is often painfully difficult for them to change their behaviours. Again, it is as though they are hypnotised into the belief that their needs are irrelevant. Even whilst acknowledging it is fine for everyone else to have needs and imperfections. For the conditioned carer their emotional needs should not exist.

Exercise 3.5 Improving Self Support

- Try taking one or two steps to support yourself better. This might include stopping to get lunch or having a coffee with a friend.

- Try to include a bit more in your conversations with those close to you about your own needs and real feelings. Showing who you are is part of becoming more truly yourself otherwise you are like a beautiful plant which hides its flowers!

How We Learn To Bury Our Feelings

- Try shifting from "perfect" to "good enough". Allow yourself to make mistakes, to get things wrong, without chastising yourself.

Jessica decided although she worked very hard she would start meeting up with some old friends to go dancing. Instead of being quite so "available" to everyone she became a bit more choosey about who she would support and started to include more of her real self in conversations. She expressed her needs more and stopped being quite so demanding with herself about getting things done.

Internal - External Support

Sadly, it has to be said that the rules above are also a strong construct within the psychology of women generally. For all the decades of feminism many women who come to see me seem to operate from them. It is not therefore surprising given this degree of emotional suppression that there is such an epidemic of obesity. But I hear you say many men are also obese!? The psychology of this is slightly different and the emotional suppression is for a different set of reasons which I will detail later.

How We Learn To Bury Our Feelings

Caring Cinderella

- "I should be there for everyone and support them"
- "I should show no needs of my own"
- "I should not show weakness

Suppress emotion "because it's not ok to reveal vulnerability"

Resentment & anger build because of not meeting needs & expressing feelings

Feel disconnected/numb in the face of difficulty or challenge from the world or others

OVER-EAT!!

How We Learn To Bury Our Feelings

Perfect Princess

Another psychological syndrome that can often be operating within the whole picture of over-eating is what I call Perfect Princess. This is not just a desire to do everything to a high standard but it includes **basing your self-worth upon this success** ie a client of mine wants to do a creative arts course but does not want to take the exam at the end because she can get nothing less than a Distinction. Consequently she is willing to give up doing the course which she will no doubt enjoy because she cannot bear to be assessed. Her self-esteem is strongly tied to her achievements and she cannot imagine simply being "good enough".

"I MUST ACHIEVE HIGHLY"

"I AM MY ACHIEVEMENTS. IF I DO NOT ACHIEVE HIGHLY I AM A FAILURE"

THIS LEAVES ME VERY ANXIOUS

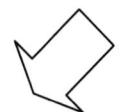

IF I DO ACHIEVE:

"WELL IT WAS TOO EASY"

IF I DO NOT ACHIEVE:

"I'M USELESS"

Exercise 3.6: Perfectionism

Notice how you treat yourself if you "make a mistake". A client of mine recently put on a big one day conference. This included speakers from around the world and hundreds of participants. The day was widely acclaimed as a great success with much positive feedback from different quarters. However, one person said they thought the buffet snack food was not really of high enough standard. My client who is addicted to perfection was mortified.

Experiment with softening towards yourself and imagining how you would view the "mistake" if this happened to a friend or one of your children. Changing perspective can often help us see how punitive we are being!

Stoic Steve lines up his Treats

Men suppress their emotions as well but generally for a different set of reasons - it may include some of the women's issues but the emphasis seems to be more:

- "I should be strong"
- "I should not express my feelings – because men don't"
- "Given how hard I work or what I have to put up with I should be allowed a few treats"
- "I want to be loved & respected but I'm damned if I'll ask for it"

How We Learn To Bury Our Feelings

Men want to be respected and loved but it's hard for them to necessarily show any of this. They expect women to intuit it and simply offer their adulation, of course! When they do not experience this love and respect men retreat further into their emotional cave and start to "treat" themselves with food/booze/drugs etc . Again, the food becomes a substitute for feeling loved. Further, it may be that they **are** loved but they do not feel this love from their partner. In this case it is more to do with the man's internal sense of loving and valuing himself. We will discuss this in more detail later in the book.

Although men function in this different way the psychological outcome is similar in that the issue still remains one of whether they can express their authentic emotional needs.

Impulsivity

The concept of "I'm entitled to a treats cos life is difficult etc...." does not just apply to men, as women will also use this type of thinking. It is closely linked to impulse control which I will now describe.

If we consider the Cycle of Awareness we start with a sensation ... become aware of it ..... we name it and start to consider our choices about what we can do. We become aware of a dry throat, we think "Oh I'm thirsty" ... **what choices do I have** ...shall I drink tea, water or juice...ok water ...we drink the water it resolves our thirst, we feel satisfied and the cycle is complete until the next need arises.

How We Learn To Bury Our Feelings

Cycle of Awareness: Left side is healthy cycle and right side unhealthy

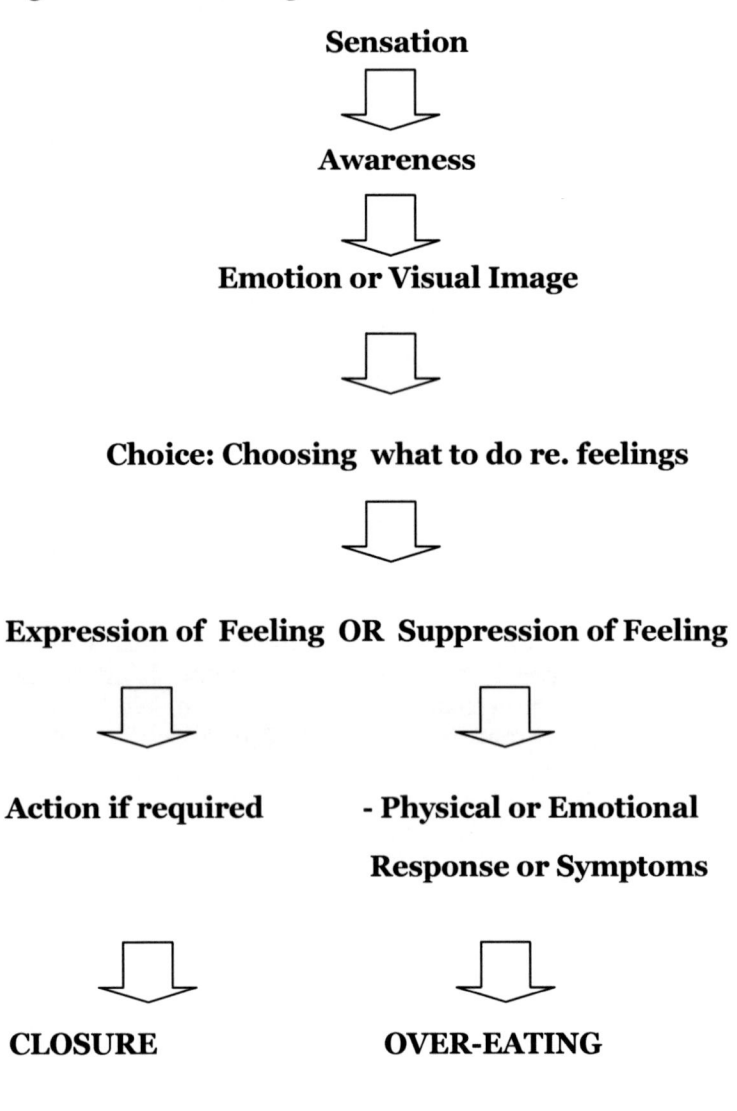

Sensation
⇩
Awareness
⇩
Emotion or Visual Image
⇩
Choice: Choosing what to do re. feelings
⇩
Expression of Feeling OR Suppression of Feeling
⇩ ⇩
Action if required   **- Physical or Emotional Response or Symptoms**
⇩ ⇩
CLOSURE   **OVER-EATING**

How We Learn To Bury Our Feelings

Where we are impulsive we usually rush from:

SENSATION................   straight to   ACTION

Completely by-passing

 REFLECTION & CHOICE!.

For example :

SENSATION............... ⟹   ACTION

I Have a:

" I NEED SOMETHING SENSATION"

EAT!

To improve our impulse control we again need to slow down our connection to the original sensation ie the " I Need Something Sensation" and allow ourselves to stay long enough with the discomfort of this to work out what we really need. If we can tolerate the discomfort of the feeling we usually find there is some emotional need that we need to resolve.

How We Learn To Bury Our Feelings

Exercise 3.7: Improving Impulse Control or Knowing What You Really Need

- Next time you find yourself automatically moving towards food, your hand is reaching for the fridge door or the biscuit tin, just pause.

- Breathe deeply

- Connect with your body. Become aware of the sensations in your body

- Consider what sort of day you have had? Is there anything upsetting or depressing you.? Are you anxious about something? Is there someone you need to speak to?

- Imagine the previous 12 or 24 hours as a graph depicting your emotions. What has happened? What were the peaks and troughs and of course where does that leave you emotionally?

- If you cannot access this information by thinking try writing down how you feel. Give yourself a few moments to reflect!

- Try to connect with what you really need emotionally. You may need to go for a walk, talk to a friend, express your irritation, cry, get a hug.

- If having done this you know you are hungry then let your hand continue on its journey to the food!

- If not find some way to act which will meet your REAL need. Consider your options for how you gain closure on whatever the **emotional issue happens to be.**

How We Learn To Bury Our Feelings

Impulse control is less about saying "Thou Shalt Not" than slowing down your automatic reaction enough to be able to experience some degree of choice.

So stoic Steve feels disrespected or un-loved. He cannot express any of this other than maybe getting stressed or angry. This pushes his partner or colleagues away which just makes him feel more unlovable. Tony goes home at night and thinks "I work really hard, I do all of this and nobody appreciates it so really I deserve a treat. Tony starts to over eat. He soon pushes away the logic of treating himself and automatically moves from feeling empty (the Sensation) to reaching out for that big warm treat (Action) which will cover over the "I Need Something Sensation".

Working with Steve I might encourage him to slow down and connect with the sensation just before he eats. I'd encourage him to imagine a graph of his mood in the six hours leading up to over-eating. Who said what to who, how did he feel about this, what would he want to say to anyone regarding any of this? If it's a long term ongoing issue it might relate to something he's sad or unhappy about which rather than being an everyday problem simply hangs over him. Again I'd encourage him to express this in the present either by saying something to me, imagining speaking to the person or writing to them. Alternatively I would encourage him to speak to the person in question. If this is not possible to start to explore why he is in an apparently very negative relationship with someone. The essence of the work would be to move from holding feelings in to expressing and possibly taking action.

Conclusion

Holding our feelings in arises because of old rules or the fear of conflict. Holding the energy in leads to us blocking our emotional energy. We become exhausted, depressed and have a sense of powerlessness. The following diagrams describe the energy dynamics of retroflection. Only by finding ways to express how we feel can we begin to regain a sense of control and actually recover a sense of energy and vitality.

Exercise 3.8 "Sitting on Things!"

Notice what happens to your energy if you "sit" on something. Notice how your energy changes when you express your feelings and how your energy is affected when you actually resolve the situation. Notice how your energy returns when you have expressed or dealt with something. Try to commit to expressing how you feel and concluding things

Clearly, there are times when I need to retroflect or not express myself. Choicefully deciding to withhold something though is very different to being on a default mechanism which means I swallow my emotion down. Not telling my ageing mother I have to go for medical tests seems like a kind withhold and therefore a choiceful choice. Once I have the test results I can decide what I will tell her. Not telling her I cannot phone her every day because I'm afraid of hurting her seems like a suppression of emotion which will end up causing me resentment rather than taking a deep breath and being honest with her.

The Energy Dynamics of Assertion

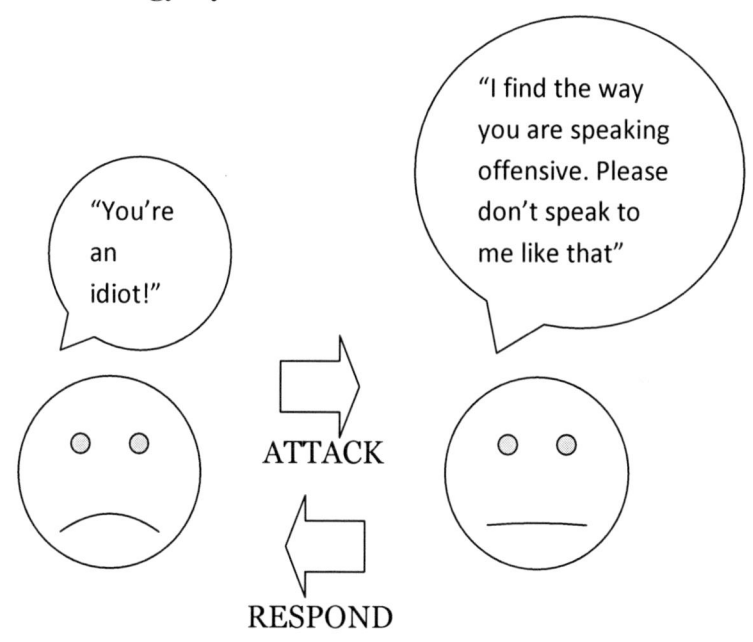

"You're an idiot!"

"I find the way you are speaking offensive. Please don't speak to me like that"

ATTACK

RESPOND

Ex.1.

In this first example someone says or does something which effects us negatively. We respond assertively by naming and questioning what they are doing. Energetically we pass the energy back to the perpetrator.

How We Learn To Bury Our Feelings

The Energy Dynamics of Suppressing Emotion

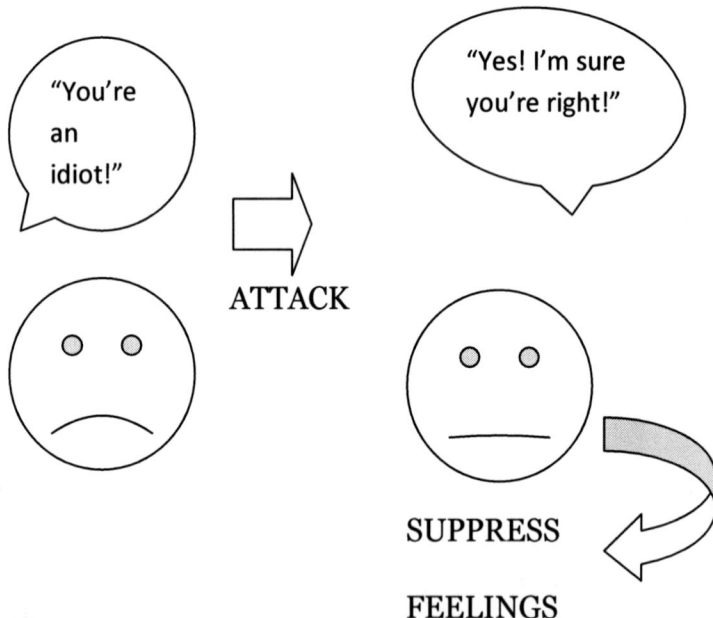

"You're an idiot!"

"Yes! I'm sure you're right!"

ATTACK

SUPPRESS FEELINGS

Ex.2

In this example someone says or does something which effects us negatively. If we do not respond then the only place for the negative energy of the comment to go is inside. We turn the energy against ourselves. This then becomes a block to the free flow of our emotional energy. We feel tired, heavy, depressed and possibly attack ourselves because we did not stand up to the offensive remark.

How We Learn To Bury Our Feelings

Undoing Suppressed Emotion

To recover from this we need to:

Finds ways to express how we feel:

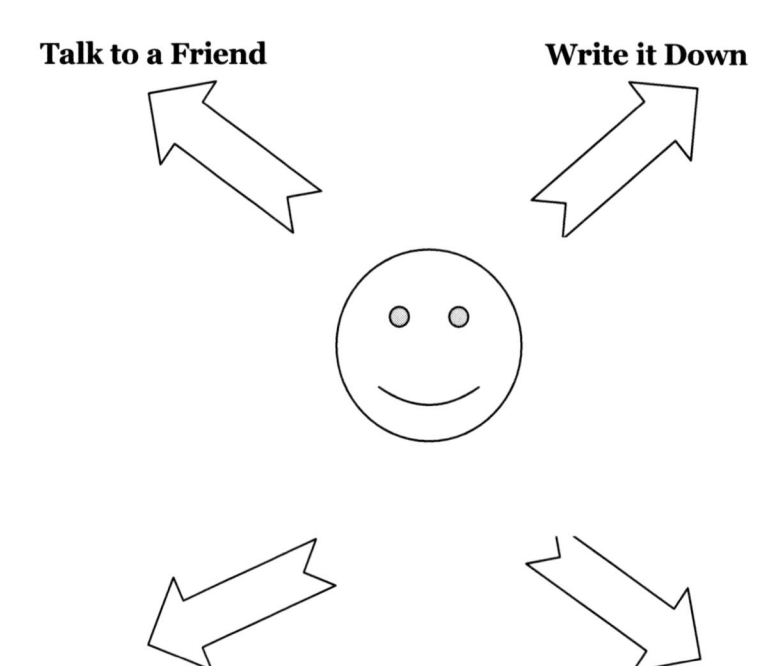

Talk to a Friend　　　　　　**Write it Down**

Talk to the person concerned　　　　**Draw a picture of how you feel**

How We Learn To Bury Our Feelings

Clients who over-eat tend to be chronic supressors of emotion. They hold their response back for fear of conflict, hurting the other, becoming enraged or becoming too visible. Learning to respond and express emotions appropriately will help you to move through the endless cycle of your emotions without becoming stuck in the negativity of retroflection.

Summary

In this chapter we have looked at:

- The importance of affection and love in shaping the brain.
- Family Rules relating to feelings & emotions. Considering the top three rules which govern your emotional life
- How suppressing emotions leads directly to over-eating
- Family control mechanisms in relation to emotions.
- Internal Control Mechanisms .How the control mechanisms in family life become internalised and we automatically control our own emotional life
- Letter to parents
- Caring Cinderella & learning to support myself

How We Learn To Bury Our Feelings

- Internal & External Support
- Stoic Steve and how men suppress emotions and "treat" themselves.
- Impulsivity + impulse control
- The energy dynamics of emotional suppression

Chapter 4

Avoiding Feelings & Over-Eating

In Chapter Three we discussed the process of burying feelings. Pushing feelings down and eating to cover up the numb-empty feeling. In this chapter we will look at another great strategy for dealing with emotions. Avoiding feelings.

I have many high achieving clients who do this. They constantly keep themselves very busy. Moving from one activity to the next. This is of course easy especially for women who can work hard all day and then go home and be busy around the house and with the demands of their families. This can affect women without families as well because the activity is moved to their social life. One client I have has a very demanding job and then social engagements every evening of the week. Her social diary is as full and varied as her work diary. This allows her to effectively ignore her internal life until of course it comes crashing in on her to remind her that "You can run but you can't hide!". Of course at this point she will collapse and become very depressed and incapable of functioning.

Usually if you start to explore compulsive "busyness" you discover that the person is either running away from feelings or that there was a very strong family injunction or

Avoiding Feelings & Over-Eating

a modelling by parents to work hard. Whichever, it tends to amount to the same thing as the rule about "working hard" will often result in a family where there is less attention to the emotional life of its members.

The imperative to work hard can arise from different sources:

"Our religion encourages us to work hard…. "the devil makes work for idle hand etc".

A generalised worry or resentment about money:

"If we don't work hard something bad will happen""I'm not having you sit around while I work so hard…"

Doing Mode vs Being Mode

At the heart of the ideas above is an interesting concept that emphasises the importance of doing over being, this often becomes what I call Doing Mode and Being Mode.

DOING MODE	**BEING MODE**
Value placed on:	*Value placed on:*
Achievements	The person in themselves
Working	
Financial Worth	Qualities rather than achievements
Material Possessions	Living in the present – the current experience
Planning for the future – the experience to come	Intuition -creativity
Analysis - rationality	

Avoiding Feelings & Over-Eating

Later, in this book in Chapter 9 you will find exercises on Mindfulness. These exercises encourage not only a way to calm your mind but also a way to help you let go of Doing Mode and move into Being Mode. Clearly to function well we need to be able to access both ways of operating.

Many people are brought up to view themselves and their world via Doing Mode. People and experiences including the experience of the self are assessed via this mode. The whole of our culture tends to emphasise this analytic rational way of dealing with the world. Clearly it can produce many benefits and yet if that is all we are then it can start to generate considerable unhappiness as has become apparent by the levels of depression which are reported throughout the "Developed" World. This mode generates endless comparison with others, ie who's achieved what, who's got what, with the consequence that we never feel enough. Mass advertising constantly and consciously fuels this desire to acquire. To be a good citizen we must consume!!

Developing acceptance of who we are and what we have whilst striving to improve for ourselves seems to generate greater happiness. Allow yourself to develop both ways of functioning and move between them trying to incorporate more being within the doing.

Doing...............Being

What I mean is that as we develop mindfulness we can be both busy but also present and attentive to the moment of our experience. Becoming more aware of our body and it's sensations we can become more skilful about taking rest or a few moments to relax within a busy day.

Avoiding Feelings & Over-Eating

A very harassed health worker came to see me recently. She was highly stressed but still just managing to work. When I described "Doing & Being" to her she became very cross and said:

"I don't have time for all this nonsense I have got a lot of work to do and many people are dependent upon me!!"

She looked so cross I thought she might hit me and I pondered that maybe she was right!! Anyway, I persevered and asked her whether she might be able to try some simple deep breathing exercises to slow her down and help control her irritability.

"What breathe in front of an office of other people!!" She sounded hugely affronted. Finally, we agreed that she could take short breaks and go outside to practise her breathing, slowing and being!! The following week she came back far sweeter tempered and said:

"You know I've started doing what you suggested and whilst it's still a very busy place I do feel a lot better, more like my old self and more in control".

If we become overly attached to Doing we often lose not only our equanimity but our sense of our real self as this lady suggests.

Avoiding feelings can take a variety of forms, the first, as we have discussed, is to simply fill your life with many things you convince yourself you have to do. Other forms of avoidance include:

Humour – joking to avoid any meaningful contact with others or yourself. This would include an ironic stance about life; being sceptical or sarcastic about anything to do

Avoiding Feelings & Over-Eating

with feelings. Are you allowed to treat yourself and your emotional life with respect?

Exercise 4.1: Humour

Notice if when you are in a social or work group you tend to play the joker. When other people say something serious you make light of it or always see the funny side. Try being aware of this tendency and then experiment with not doing it. Be aware of the effect this has? Initially you may feel more uncomfortable but notice if you respond seriously what happens to the conversation. Humour is great but if you always default to being jokey or ironic you may miss interesting things about yourself and others!

Avoiding silence in conversations. Many people find silence uncomfortable and rush to fill it during a conversation yet this may mean you miss the most interesting or intimate part of the dialogue.

Exercise 4.2: Dealing with Silence

Notice if you feel un-easy with silence in conversation. Experiment with allowing what was previously a tiny pause and see if you can breathe deeply and let it run a little longer. Be aware of what happens when you do not leap in to fill the gap. Often the other person will say something or move the conversation to a deeper level which is not possible if every space is filled. Experiment just at the edge of your comfort zone and see what you learn.

Eye Contact

Avoiding eye contact is another way of deflecting from connecting with other people. If you tend to look away or look down a lot try, as with the silence, just holding the contact a little bit longer than you would usually. Enormous amounts of communication goes on through eye contact. If you miss it, well you miss it!

Exercise 4.3: Eye Contact

Try holding eye contact a little more or a little longer than usual. As you do so breathe and try affirming yourself with a simple affirmation such as" It's fine for me to be here" or " I am equal with this person". Eye contact can be intrusive so do not over-do it. Notice how you feel as you hold more eye contact than previously.

Avoiding Being Alone

Clients who struggle with their own feelings or sense of themselves often go to great lengths to avoid spending time alone. Being alone has different meanings for different people. For some it seems to indicate that they have failed because they are alone. As though the action is happening elsewhere and they are missing it! Somehow being alone can never be enough – they need the affirmation of the other person's presence to feel fully alive. For other people it is more that when they are alone their real feelings start to surface and they do not like the feelings or themselves.

Avoiding Feelings & Over-Eating

Part of coming to terms with being alone is the acceptance that we are essentially alone; this is a part of being human. We are not born as a collective we are born as a unique and single individual. Learning to live with ourselves requires that we be in good relation with ourselves. If we have internalised a negative or disparaging inner voice then being alone will be a struggle. A bit like spending the evening with a critical friend who insists we should be living our life differently. To live with ourselves happily requires a process of befriending and encouraging ourselves; learning to be our own best friend. This does not mean that there is no discrimination about what is good or bad for us but rather that our inner voice develops more kindness and compassion

Exercise 4.4: Being Alone

Reflect on how you feel about being fundamentally alone in the world. Does being in this world leave you feeling angry? Some clients have said they are angry because they had no choice in being born; that it was a process beyond their control. Other people say when they reflect on their aloneness they feel anxious. Do you have as much right to be on the planet as other people? If not, why not?

Try saying the following statements, whether you believe them or not:

"I choose to be born and to be present in my life here, today with all its pleasures and all its difficulties"

And then:

"I choose to accept my aloness in the world and see it as a challenge to live as well as I can given this fact"

Avoiding Feelings & Over-Eating

When I think of these issues I often think of the natural world and the huge variety of plants and animals each of which has its own unique place within the ecosystem. I imagine a monkey rather dolefully saying:

"Of course I never wanted to be a monkey. I always wanted to be a tiger. Much faster and more glamorous" or like the paranoid android Marvin in The Hitchhikers Guide to the Galaxy "Life? Don't talk to me about life!".

These are all forms of passive aggression. What I mean is that they involve a quietly angry denial of the actual reality ie "I am a monkey or I am a robot" . Now, how do I make this a good experience? Regularly stating that you choicefully accept the conditions of your life gives you a real opportunity to be with that condition and either accept it or if necessary change it. Our being alone in the world is a fundamental given and in the end I either accept it or will in some way be crushed by it!

Authentic vs In-authentic

A client said to me recently, "I feel as though my inside and my outside are two completely different people. There's what I present and what feel inside. I feel as though I want to learn to marry them up"

Her instinct was a good one. Jane was raised in a very religious and traditional family where it was demanded she behave in certain ways. Over time she got so used to playing a part that she actually lost who she truly was. This happened so completely that she became scared of her emotions. Her natural feelings felt wrong to her.

Avoiding Feelings & Over-Eating

Jane through the demands of her family had spent so long deflecting from her feelings that she had developed a strong external facade. At the point she came to me she had virtually become the facade. There was just a little glimmer of the real her, who felt how she was living was wrong.

Working over time I encouraged and supported her to acknowledge her feelings and begin to stand up to the internalised belief structure which caused her so many problems. This mixture of assertion in relation to the old rules and developing compassion towards the self that was so buried enabled her to rapidly start re-discovering herself. Jane started with very small steps to more authentically assert who she was. Expressing a different point of view or asserting a need regarding something allowed her to learn that the world would not come crashing down if she became more authentic.

Exercise 4.5 Being Authentic!

We often struggle with being fully authentic because of our fear that we will be disliked or rejected. I often think of in-authenticity as a person who is just two dimensional and black and white then beginning to let their colours show. As the colour seeps through so they become more three dimensional, vivid and alive. They are living an authentic life!

Consider how authentic you are? How much of your life are you playing a role? Are you like Jane disconnecting the inner you from the outer you? Do you speak in clichés or do you allow yourself to express what you truly believe?

Avoiding Feelings & Over-Eating

Like Jane notice where you withhold yourself and begin to allow yourself to reveal more of who you are. This could include expressing opinions which are contrary to others or expressing needs or emotions. Notice what happens when you do this. Some people may not like it if you become more expressive. Notice what happens to you when you are more expressive

If I want to be more authentically myself I have to accept that some people may not like this. Again, I will need to drop the need for their approval.

Deciding whether you are going to live in a more authentic way is clearly a big challenge. If you have experienced disapproval, the threat of violence or violence itself this may have strongly conditioned you to hide your real self. Yet, the hiding or suppression of your true self is a core part of your over-eating. The more you can freely express who and how you are the less you will feel emotionally "blocked" and that the only resolution is to eat.

Authenticity and Compassion

Clients who start to become more emotionally expressive often report two things:

- "I feel better expressing myself"
- "I feel that I'm behaving badly"

If you start to express yourself more fully you will also find that you need to over-eat less. As you eat less you will tend to experience your emotions more fully. This can be quite alarming if you are used to muting your feelings.

Clients who are working through the Love Myself Slim approach often come in at this stage and report that they are having more disagreements with people, conflicts are occurring which did not previously happen. Clients often feel they are going backwards and that they have become "bad". If they appear reporting this I reassure them they are right on track!! If you become more authentically yourself then this means you should be stating your opinions, needs and wants more clearly. This in turn will create a reaction which may leave you feeling you are "bad" rather than the "good" compliant person who previously agreed with everyone.

Clearly you have a choice. If you become more expressive this will create more waves and you may upset people. The issue then becomes for me the way in which you deliver your authenticity. Essentially this becomes about a balance between authenticity and compassion:

Authenticity

vs

Compassion

Avoiding Feelings & Over-Eating

Example: Authenticity & Compassion

If I want to stay emotionally healthy and not over-eat I need to live authentically and express my feelings and yet equally I want to treat other people well and not become some sort of egocentric monster. I therefore need to balance my sense of my authentic needs with a sense of compassion for others. This is not about defaulting to taking care of others but rather being wise about my own needs and offering other people what I reasonably can.

Susan was asked for feedback by a colleague Sarah, who had been reprimanded by their boss. Susan checked that she did want feedback and then said that at times she experienced Sarah as patronising and arrogant and that this was possibly the way customers experienced her. Sarah received the feedback without much comment but later became offended and Susan then felt bad that she had been "so authentic". When we looked at this Susan had both checked if Sarah wanted feedback and again later had asked if Sarah was ok with hearing difficult feedback. She had delivered the feedback as calmly and gently as she felt she could whilst being frank with Sarah. In terms of our discussion Susan had been both authentic and compassionate.

Exercise 4.6 Authenticity & Compassion

Think of a current situation where you would like to express yourself more authentically. Think of what you really want to communicate and then how you can do this whilst being compassionate to the other person. If you struggle with this discuss it with a friend to see if they can help you find an appropriate way to convey your feelings. When you have a form of words try experimenting with actually saying them out loud to see how they sound.

Avoiding Feelings & Over-Eating

Needs Review

To establish a clear boundary regarding authenticity and compassion I need to review my life and decide what are the fundamental things I need to be healthy, happy and well. This will enable me to establish some ground rules about who and how I am. So, I might decide I need to eat certain foods, exercise a certain amount have enough input from things which relax me like friends, hobbies or cultural pursuits.

Exercise 4.7 Needs Review

What is a good diet for me?

What exercise keeps me feeling well?

How much exercise do I need each week to feel well?

What do I need from my relationship? Can I ask for this?

Am I happy with work? If not what can I change?

How much socialising do I need? Am I getting this?

What activities do I enjoy outside work? Am I getting enough of these?

Do I have enough space? Do I have too much?

Avoiding Feelings & Over-Eating

Commitment

Having decided what keeps you happy, healthy and well you need to commit to getting enough of these elements within your life. Become more assertive about maintaining these activities. Of course some weeks you may need to be flexible but if you keep flexing you will end up meeting everyone else's needs!

Conclusion

In this chapter we have explored how we can deflect from or avoid our real emotions. We can do this through being hyper-busy, through humour, avoiding silence, avoiding eye contact, avoiding being alone and through irritability. All of these ways of behaving tend to prioritise Doing Mode and prevent us from operating from what I call Being Mode. We are therefore less authentic because we hide or suppress our real needs and feelings. In order to change this we need to commit to the value of authenticity both as a good way to live and also because it is more healthy emotionally. Of course to do this requires quite a lot of courage because we risk being disliked yet if we are not authentic then we become "emotionally constipated" and yet again are more likely to over-eat as a consequence

Summary

In this chapter we discussed:

- Deflection & being busy
- Doing Mode and Being Mode

Avoiding Feelings & Over-Eating

- Humour as avoidance
- Eye Contact
- Silence
- Being Alone
- Authentic vs In-authentic
- Authenticity & Compassion
- Needs Review

Chapter Five
These Emotions Are Nothing To Do With Me!

In the previous chapter we were considering how we can deflect or avoid our emotional life by being busy. Also, how we may use humour to divert from our authentic inner life and its expression in the world. In this chapter I want to explore another mechanism by which we prevent ourselves connecting, what Jane called, our inner and outer selves. This mechanism where we "project" our emotions onto another person is called Projection.

Understanding how we avoid our emotions can help us to express them. As previously described, improving our ability to be emotionally expressive rather than emotionally repressive will greatly reduce our need to over-eat.

Example

Gary feels useless about his abilities because his father always criticized him. It is hard for him to acknowledge how he feels so when colleagues or friends make small mistakes

These Emotions Are Nothing To Do With Me

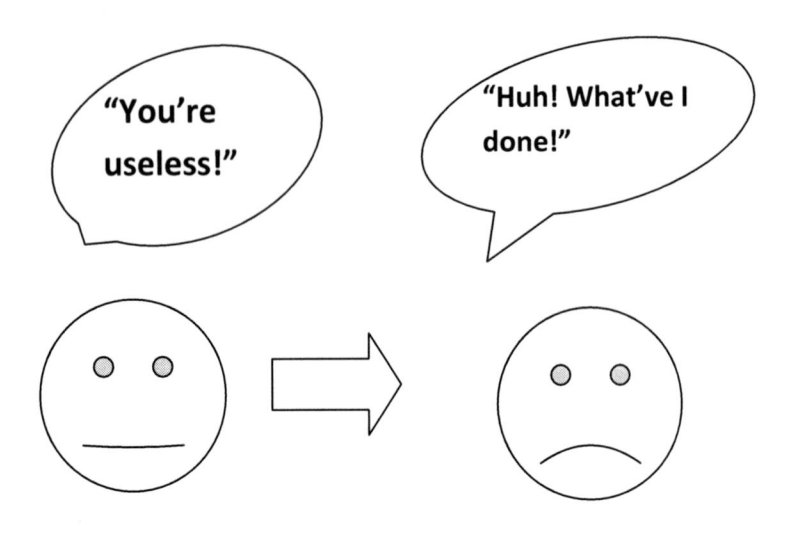

"You're useless!" → "Huh! What've I done!"

A.　　　　　Projection　　　　　**B.**

Person A "I feel useless but cannot acknowledge this because for some reason it is too difficult" So, "I'm fine you are useless

Person B: " I do not understand why I am being attacked"

Gary will be very critical. He therefore projects his unacknowledged feelings onto other people.

Sally grew up in a family which had very little money. Now she is in a good job with a good salary. Without realising it she is very anxious about money and often mean because of this. However, in a bar with friends she is very critical of a particular friend who has genuinely forgotten their wallet and doesn't buy a round. She projects her difficulty with money onto someone else

These Emotions Are Nothing To Do With Me

The central theme with projection is the person's lack of awareness of their own emotional life and their tendency to "put their emotions on other people".

To establish if you are doing this try the following exercise:

Exercise 5.1 Projection

- Notice the degree to which you tend to criticise and blame other people. Other people obviously do make mistakes but if we tend to find fault in others it may be that we are not acknowledging these issues within ourselves, like Gary and Sally.

- Think of a criticism you've made of someone recently "Oh she's so stuck-up". Check your own capacity for being stuck-up. When were you last superior? It may be true that this person is "stuck-up" and it may be an expression of an aspect of yourself.

- Look at a painting with a friend and imagine what the emotions of the artist were as s/he made the painting. Using exactly the same language now express these emotions as your own. " I feel....". We cannot know what an artist or composer is really feeling and part of the pleasure of the arts is that we tend to project ourselves into the artistic product. All the words you used about the painting were actually yours and the emotions were primarily about you! See what our friend felt. This can be particularly revealing if you do it with an abstract painting as the interpretation we make can be more varied between people.

These Emotions Are Nothing To Do With Me

Irritability & Defensiveness

Another form of deflection from experiencing ourselves and other people is irritability itself. Being grouchy or cronky can become great way to prevent yourself feeling other emotions or allowing other people to give you feedback about yourself. We may have developed a rather spiky persona or facade as a way to keep emotions at bay.

I was recently in hospital awaiting some minor surgery in a bay of other patients also awaiting procedures. One man came in and from the beginning he found fault with everything: the nurses were too slow, the service was terrible the food they were proposing to serve later was all wrong:

"What do you mean you're going to give me sandwiches! Do you not understand I have a very sore throat. I need soup. Soup, I said! Why can't you understand a perfectly reasonable request!"

Yes, it was a bit like an episode of Fawlty Towers! All of this was directed at a very friendly and professionally competent nursing team. He then got onto his mobile and was screaming at a mechanic who was giving him some bad news about his car. His irritability struck me as a complete defence against the anxiety of having his medical procedure. Later in the day when his medical issues had been resolved he left and very meekly told the nurses, somewhat to their surprise, how wonderful they had all been! Rather than be able to experience his anxiety about the procedure he had found fault with everything and in a sense projected his anxiety out onto the world as a fault finding attack.

These Emotions Are Nothing To Do With Me

Projection & Over-Eating

In the same way that we can interrupt our emotions by rules from our past, or by deflecting into "busyness" so we can project our emotions onto others and effectively disown how we feel. If I have little connection with my sensations or emotions it is easy to push my feelings away and out onto the world:

"It's your fault I feel this way"

Typically, clients who over-eat tend to project onto the world less that people are bad than that they are better than them. In this way they disown their own power. How does this work?

These Emotions Are Nothing To Do With Me

"You are so big & powerful!"

"Hey! If you want to see me that way! Fine! Bring it on!"

POWER

A.

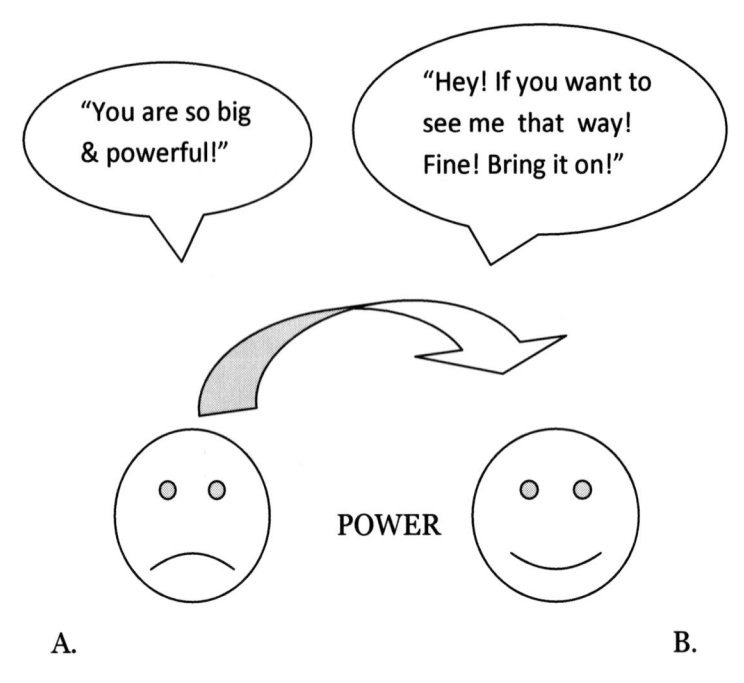

" I couldn't possibly imagine any power so I'll give it all to you"

B.

"I don't know why you are doing this but I enjoy it!"

Of course having set up this dynamic Person A inherits the consequences: see over

These Emotions Are Nothing To Do With Me

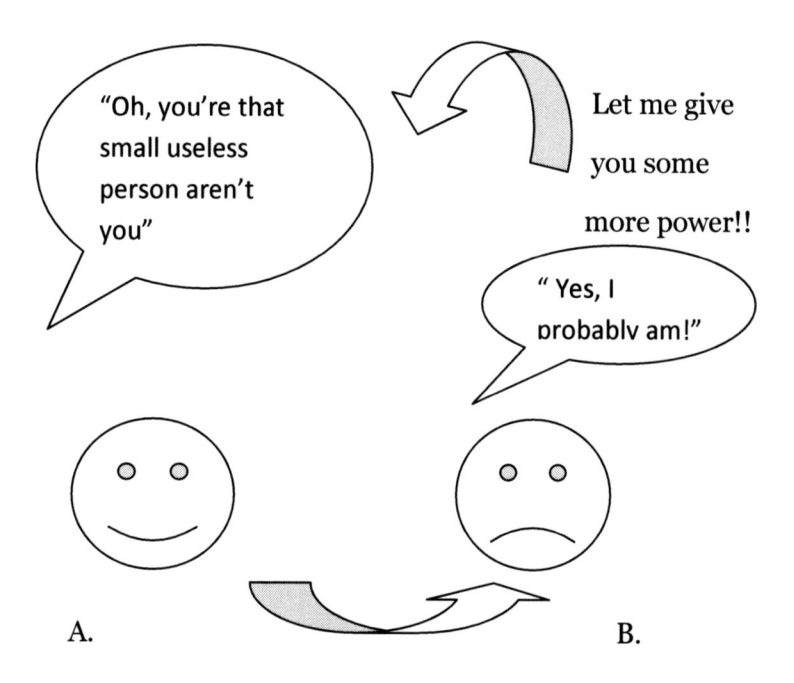

"Oh, you're that small useless person aren't you"

Let me give you some more power!!

" Yes, I probably am!"

A.　　　　　　　　　B.

POWER OVER

Having been given the power it is not surprising if B enjoys this feeling and then comes to see it as their right to enjoy their power or authority over A. This could only happen because A cannot believe or will not believe that they can have their own power. They project this power onto B who then of course enjoys it to the full and quite probably ends up abusing or disrespecting A in some form

Projecting our own feelings onto other people can be a great way to avoid facing our own negative or darker feelings. By noticing our criticisms and judgements of others we can learn about what we may really be feeling about ourselves.

These Emotions Are Nothing To Do With Me

Whose Life is it Anyway!

Have you ever felt like an observer or an actor in your own life? We have probably all had this sensation at some time of stepping outside ourselves and noticing how we behave. For some clients this can become a routine way of experiencing themselves. Sheila says:

"I do not really feel fully alive! It's as though I watch myself all the time. As though I see myself as others do! I feel it makes me more cautious in interacting with my friends and colleagues. I would love to feel as though I'm at the centre of my own life and that I can be spontaneous and free"

Sheila is experiencing another way in which we interrupt our awareness of our emotions . What I call The Observer position. The developing child in this situation has usually been taught that their reactions, thoughts or emotions are in some way not acceptable to their parents. The child's creative response to this is to live slightly outside their own experience and observe or monitor their reactions and behaviour. Whilst this makes them safer as a child from disapproval it can become a habitual way of relating to themselves and to the world. The image that springs to mind of this is of a desktop icon on a computer where the icon has been slightly moved and is not fully aligned with itself. The icon only becomes functional when it is aligned and this is of course true of the individual who needs to learn to become more integrated into themselves.

These Emotions Are Nothing To Do With Me

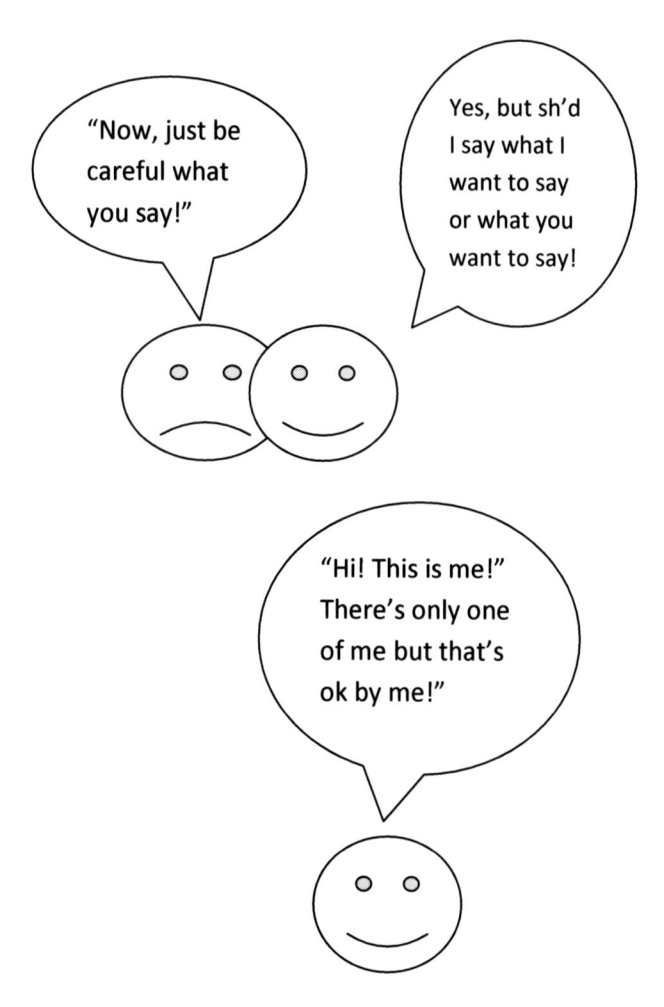

Exercise 5.2: Watching Yourself

Become aware of the degree to which you "self-monitor". Notice the amount of background commentary you make on your own behaviour. Sometimes this can be helpful and supportive but if you do it a lot it may be because you are overly anxious about "getting things wrong".

These Emotions Are Nothing To Do With Me

Encourage yourself to be more accepting of your responses and reactions to the world. Even if you have a different view to others. Develop your own personal mantra:

"It's fine for me to have my own emotions and views about things" or

"I fully accept myself exactly how I am!"

Learning to re-integrate back into yourself will require you to regularly remind yourself that it is fine to be you. If you think how long you have been living in this way you will need to definitely work at encouraging a new attitude within yourself.

Exercise 5.3: Embodied Affirmation

You will also need to support these affirmations with slow, deep breathing to help incorporate this new information into your body. When we are learning something new it needs to be not only in our heads but in our feelings and importantly in our body. As you vocalise the affirmations above breathe and imagine drawing them deeper and deeper into your body. Draw the affirmation down into your lungs and imagine this new information entering your blood stream like the oxygen you just breathed in. Picture the affirmation circulating and entering every cell in your body. Imagine becoming a living embodiment of the affirmation:

"I fully accept myself exactly how I am!"

If you have got used to living in this slightly detached way you may also need to re-commit to living your own life. Until you make this commitment your life will be like a sailing boat with no rudder that simply gets blown around by the passing winds. As with the ideas in Chapter Two regarding family rules you may need to challenge some of these rules

These Emotions Are Nothing To Do With Me

regarding how you were supposed to behave. Look back at Chapter 2 for more details on how to do this.

Finally, living more fully in ourselves requires that we live in the Here & Now. Most of my clients who come to see me tend to live mostly in the past or the future or a mixture of the two. They remember bad things that happened or they are anxious about things to come. Most of us do this most of the time yet of course the past and the future are a fantasy which we create in our minds. As all the philosophers and mystics down the years have said the only knowable reality is the Here & Now. The more we can ground ourselves in the moment the more alive we will be AND the safer we will feel!

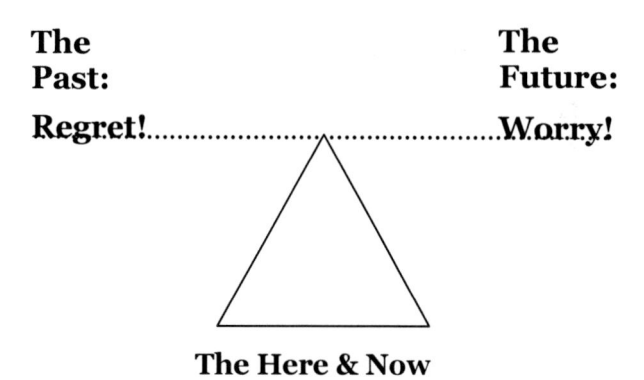

The Past: Regret! .... **The Future: Worry!**

The Here & Now

Like a seesaw we can tip backwards and forwards between worry of the future and regret of the past. It is only when we start to live predominantly in the moment of the here & now that we start to more fully experience ourselves and the

These Emotions Are Nothing To Do With Me

world. Before this our life will be more bound up with our inner fantasy life. In my experience of working with many clients who have been traumatised they predominantly live in a muddle of past terrors and future anxieties. Their recovery always involves fully embracing the present moment and the sense of safety which this brings

The Three Zones

Fritz Perls who originated Gestalt Therapy, upon which a lot of this book is based, talked about the Three Zones of Awareness. The Inner Zone contains all the sensations of the body – these are actual and knowable experiences, the Outer Zone is the world of tables, chairs, books, pictures, cars etc which are tangible things we can touch and feel. Everything else dreams, thoughts, memories, reflection are all the stuff of the Middle Zone. For Fritz, living healthily and sanely required spending much less time in the Middle Zone where we neurotically fret, ruminate and catastrophise or worry obsessively about the future. Grounding ourselves in what is actual, real and tangible can produce a major improvement in mental and physical health.

These Emotions Are Nothing To Do With Me

The Three Zones of Awareness

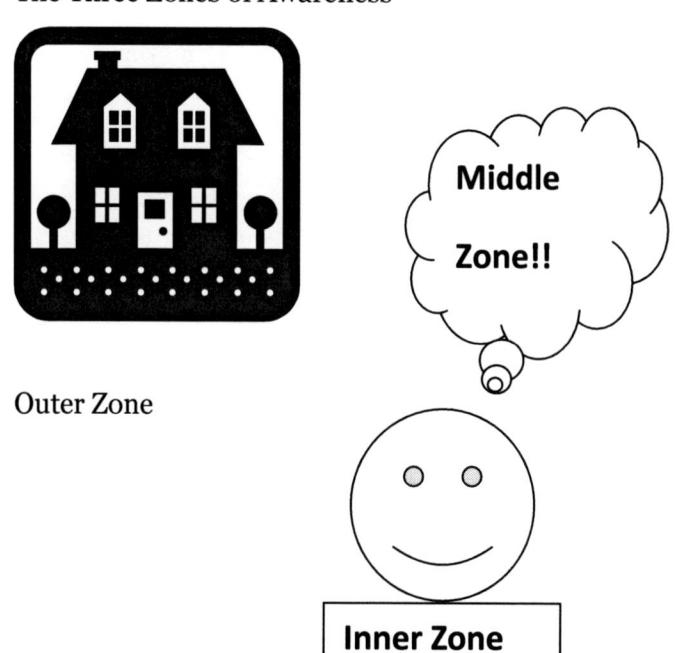

Outer Zone

Middle Zone!!

Inner Zone

Inner Zone: Sensations, body awareness

Middle Zone: Thoughts, feelings, fantasies

Outer Zone: The environment – cars houses, fields, tables, chairs , people

These Emotions Are Nothing To Do With Me

Exercise 5.4: The Three Zones

The following exercise combines both a developing awareness of the Here & Now with a sense of the three zones described above. This exercise is a foundational exercise and can be helpful whichever way you tend to block or interrupt your emotional experience.

Deepen and slow your breathing and become aware of the sensations in your body.

Inner Zone:

Notice where you are tense and holding and where you feel relaxed and soft. Maybe adjust your position as you become aware of any tensions or allow yourself to just sit with the tension. As you become aware of sensations simply say, for example:

"Here & now I am aware of the tension in my shoulder, here and now I am aware of how relaxed my stomach feels"

Middle Zone:

Move your awareness to your thoughts and emotions as you notice what you are feeling and thinking again describe them:

"Here and now I am aware of feeling sad about Sally. I notice my thoughts keep returning to her"

Outer Zone:

Move your awareness to your environment. Notice the light, the shapes, the objects, the sounds around you. As you take in your environment say:

These Emotions Are Nothing To Do With Me

"Here and now I am aware of the light falling on the table and the sound of the children playing outside"

Now mindfully move your awareness between the three zones. Be aware of the degree to which you can allow yourself to be present here and now in the moment. Notice how your thoughts and feelings may draw you away. Consider how your thoughts and feelings are an interpretation or "overlay" on your direct experiencing of the self and the world. See if you can allow yourself to simply sit with your sensations and immediate experience of the world.

When I do this exercise with clients they will often report how jumbled they initially feel with a lot of thoughts and emotions occurring and little awareness of their body or environment. As they direct their attention to the Inner and Outer Zones so they become more peaceful and a tangible sense of peace often develops in the room as though the endless chatter of their mind commenting and diverting them has been temporarily stilled.

Having learnt this exercise you can use it at any time in the future to check in with yourself. If you find your thoughts or emotions are particularly strong it may mean you either actually need to attend to something or that you use more deep breathing to help calm and slow your mind.

These Emotions Are Nothing To Do With Me

Summary

Defining Projection

Irritability & Defensiveness

Projection & Over-Eating

Egotising or Observer position

Embodying Affirmation

The Three Zones

Chapter 6

"This Body is Nothing To Do With Me Either!"

As children we are frequently set emotional problems which we learn to resolve the best way we can. We want Mummy to love us but she seems to keep finding fault with what we do. We learn to adapt to try to deliver what she wants because we want that approval so much. In doing so we lose something. We lose a part of ourselves or part of us closes down. Given we are little and have limited resources it is not surprising if we do not always resolve these emotional puzzles particularly well. Yet of course what we do as children is that..... WE DO THE BEST WE CAN!

It's often only years later when our emotional life hits the buffers that we start to wake up to the idea that the "resolution" we came to when we were six years old may not be the best resolution now. People tend to come and see therapists when the book of rules, the resolutions they have been living by cease to work. It is my job then as a therapist to try and work out what may have gone wrong. This is a bit like detective work as I try to understand the patterns that were laid down in childhood that have resulted in the person behaving the way they currently do.

"This Body is Nothing To Do With Me Either!"

So far we have explored six ways in which as children we learn to block out our emotional experience. I have left the seventh to the last because in many ways it is the toughest both for the client and the therapist!

We have explored how early family rules can cause us to think and feel in certain ways. One "resolution" to these rules can be that I choose to stop feeling and enter a state of denial. I conclude that I am someone who does not have emotions.. All the other forms of emotional adaption we have discussed still allow for some feeling. In this form the child decides that what they are exposed to from their parents is so painful or toxic that they are going to just close down. This is what I call Blanking.

When you ask a client who is de-sensitised how they feel they will be genuinely bemused. One client I had would repeatedly pause and quite obviously reflect and say "You know, I do not know how I feel".

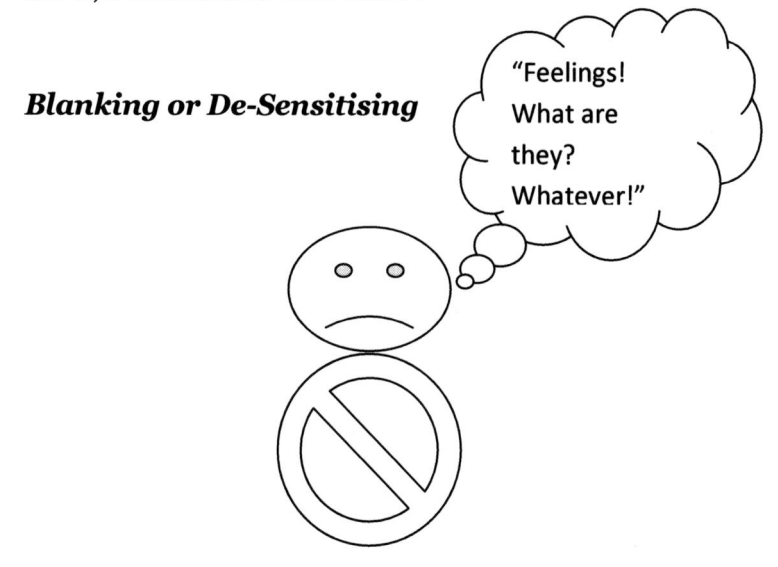

Blanking or De-Sensitising

"Feelings! What are they? Whatever!"

"This Body is Nothing To Do With Me Either!"

I worked for months with this client to slowly re-sensitise her to her own feelings. This involved challenging various old rules:

- It's not ok to have feelings
- Feelings are dangerous
- You should cope. Just get on with it.
- People with feelings are weak
- You are only strong if you show nothing
- It's ok for other people to have feelings but not me

With these clients the rules embed the emotional cutting-off. Changing is primarily about starting to feel sensations in the body. Understanding that emotions always start with a sensation of something in your body is crucial to re-connecting with your felt sense of self!

Exercise 6.1 Tuning into Sensation

Start to notice how your body is amazing at sending you all sorts of data about your reactions to people and the world. You meet Frank and your stomach goes into a knot. You meet Jill and you feel this warm fuzzy feeling!! You think about work and your chest tightens slightly you think about your niece or your grandchild and your face breaks into an automatic smile. Our body contains its own wisdom and we often spend a lot of time and often an expensive education denying its very existence. So, become more aware of your bodily reactions but especially if you are choosing something.

"This Body is Nothing To Do With Me Either!"

Take something you are making a decision about. Let's say you have three options. Be aware of what your mind says and then what your body says. In his book *Blink* Malcolm Gladwell describes how our bodies know things very rapidly and often much more accurately then our brains'.

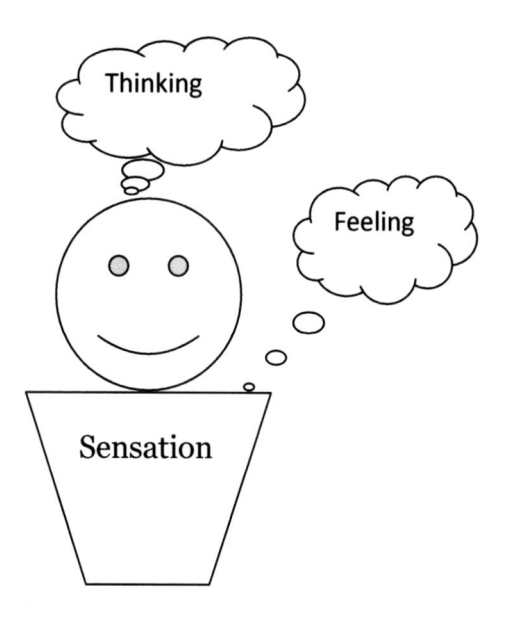

Whilst we experience feedback from ourselves in the form of thoughts, feelings and sensations people who de-sensitise tend to prioritise thinking; sensations and emotions are more difficult.

Starting to re-sensate ie to get to know your sensations and feelings requires you to re-acquaint yourself ...with yourself ...in fine detail!

"This Body is Nothing To Do With Me Either!"

Exercise 6.2 : Inner Zone

As you sit here with the book in your hands become aware of your body. Allow your attention to move through and around all your body. Notice as before where there is tension and where there is relaxation. Notice any commentary you may make regarding your body. Notice the thought and yet bring your attention back to the sensation of your body. Try to simply be with yourself as your body. As you continue to sit with yourself notice if any particular focus or figure emerges. Maybe there is a tension in your shoulder from all this reading! Simply be aware of this tension. Notice what comments, thoughts or emotions you have about your body. If the tension continues notice if there is a need developing out of the focus or figure. For example, you may become aware that your bladder is full, or that you are feeling quite cold.

For who are blanking the first stage of recovery is to really start to listen in fine detail to your body. Initially this may feel a bit strange or very strange. This is not something you are necessarily going to be aware of.. You may even be so used to this "numbing" of yourself that you are not aware of it. In my experience most people who over-eat de-sensitise a lot, almost by definition. Some clients may have this as their primary adaption to emotional contact whilst for others it may be one part of a wider picture.

As you develop your awareness start to develop a dialogue with your body. Check in on a regular basis ie "Good morning body! How are you doing?". Listen to the response. This feedback from your body is every bit as important as what your brain says. As you lead your life try to refer more to the responses of your body. All this information is available to you and yet for years you may have been filtering it out.

"This Body is Nothing To Do With Me Either!"

One client in a group I worked with became quite shocked at the suggestion that she should give equal attention to her body as to her thinking.

"But I've always taught my children, let alone myself, NOT to do that. I mean they would, I would, just become an impulsive animal!"

Interestingly she was one of the most disconnected people in the group. She was lovely and very intellectually bright but clearly divorced from any contact with her body and sensations.

This view of your body as something you have to correct and control seems to be based upon a very punitive view that makes the intellect or the brain the superior master over the wayward, inherently slothful body. Rather, my view would be that the brain and the body have their own wisdom and that we need to listen to both. Whilst I may learn to listen more clearly to the needs of my body I can still use my brain to exercise choice and decide what is ultimately healthy or right for me.

It is one thing to listen to the responses of your body yet the next stage is how you classify that information and then what you do about it. The process looks something like the diagram on the next page.

"This Body is Nothing To Do With Me Either!"

Sensation

"Empty Stomach"

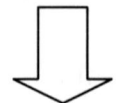

⬇

Name sensation

"Hungry"

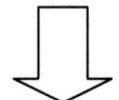

⬇

Mobilise

"Start to think about food"

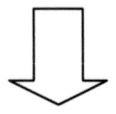

⬇

Action

Make food

"This Body is Nothing To Do With Me Either!"

Sensations to Needs

For someone who is desensitised they may completely ignore the "Empty stomach" sensations and for example work a long day without eating anything. As the sensation (empty stomach) comes more into focus (hunger) and evolves into a need (food) all sorts of old rules, whether conscious or not may start to come into play:

"That's just your body – use your will power you do not need to eat"

"Why look after your self – no one else did!"

"You're not worth it!" ie taking care of yourself

"Who said life was comfortable?"

So, there may be an over-riding sense that you generally ignore your body – this is a Master Rule ie a very key and deep rule which you may have lived with for years. You may well not be aware of this sort of rule as it is often quite deeply buried and "locked" as described in Chapter 2 on Rules. This may then be surrounded by a sub-menu of other rules such as those above. These all inter-lock to create a neat rubrics cube which essentially maintains you in believing it is fine not to take real care of yourself. Quite simply not eating all day is not good for you!

Become familiar with the sensations in your body and then the needs which arise out of these sensations. This process is going on all day every day. As you become more conscious of this process notice how you interrupt the meeting of your needs. "Oh I'm ok, I went five hours ago!!".

"This Body is Nothing To Do With Me Either!"

Developing your ability to listen to these small or not so small signals from your body may seem unimportant yet they are the building blocks of starting to move from being blocked off and disconnected from the authentic you!! To a large degree you are a composite of all these emerging needs and disowning them means you disown yourself

To summarise, to re-sensate or regain your sense of your body you need to:

1. Tune in and listen to the sensations in your body – use deep slow breathing to help with this.

2. Start to name the sensations: develop a vocabulary of your body "Oh there goes my stomach…tightening up"

3. Identify if there is a need, arising from the sensation: I'm hungry"

4. Decide if there is anything you want to do about this need: i.e, I'll make some food"

5. Notice how you may undermine or minimise the need by old rules: "You can eat tonight i.e over-eat"

In addition to needs arising from sensation we may also experience as described before, emotions and images arising from sensations

"This Body is Nothing To Do With Me Either!"

Exercise 6.3 Sensation-Image-Thought-Feeling

Focus your attention on your body. Become aware of sensations in your body. Notice whether there is:

A physical need attached to this sensation.....feeling thirsty, hungry, cold etc

An emotion related to the sensation.... sad, anxious, happy

An image attached to the sensation... "When I have that sensation I picture....."

A thought attached to this sensation: "I think I'll go to London tomorrow". A mixture of two or more of the above.

Try to start making it a regular part of your day that you check in with your body, noticing the information it gives you regarding needs, emotions and images. Regard this as important information from yourself. Stop filtering this information out but rather use it to help make choices in you life. This can apply whether you are deciding what to have for lunch or which job to go for.

A crucial part of re-sensating or getting to know your body and its sensations is being able to decipher the information from your body. What does it mean when my stomach tightens? Why do I always picture a certain street when I get that sensation? Why do I feel sad when I have that sensation? To fully engage with yourself you have to be willing to "listen" in much greater detail to the information from your body. Notice how your old emotional habits kick in to get you to deny, disown or discard your experience. Changing the old habit of pushing your emotional/sensation reactions away will take time.

"This Body is Nothing To Do With Me Either!"

Try developing a vocabulary for your body-mind to more clearly capture your personal experience ie when my tummy tightens that means I'm scared, when I swallow that means I am angry, when I have a headache that often means I'm tense or angry. Naming your experience will take you half way to being able to manage it.

Summary

- Defining Blanking
- Exercise: Sensation
- Exercise Inner Zone
- Sensation to Needs
- Sensation-Image-Thought-Feeling

Chapter 7

Shame

In the previous chapter we explored the issue of blanking or blocking out your emotions. When we de-sensitize there is often a particular emotional pattern underlying this behaviour; this is known as shame. Although clients who over-eat may have widely varying childhoods the experience of shame is frequently a common theme. In this circumstance the experience of parental criticism goes far beyond feeling criticized about something; the child will feel that as a person they are inadequate or incompetent. This is not about what they do but who they feel they are.

Understanding if you are shame-based as a person can be very helpful as you find new ways to support yourself . Even if this is not a core part of how you function clients who over-eat often refer to shame regarding their eating patterns or body image. Firstly, I want to simply describe shame. Notice if you relate to any of these descriptions.

What is Shame

Gary Yontef describes shame as individuals experiencing one or more of the following:

Shame

- In addition to feeling weak or incompetent they may feel defective, stupid, boring, "not enough". These can be emotions and or thoughts.

- Regarding oneself as disgusting, repugnant to others, loathsome, untouchable, unwanted, a bother or nuisance, not a gift.

- Being un- entitled and unworthy of respect, belonging, success, love, comfort, hence feeling more shame and guilt when good things happen.

- Feeling one's privacy painfully violated by being seen by others, the eyes of the other becoming a glaring spotlight that leaves one feeling transparent, that one's secrets are exposed to the public glare and naked and vulnerable to contempt one believes is well-deserved.

Recently, when working with a client who over-eats she was describing an experience at home I said "The word shame, keeps coming to mind". She started to cry and said:"You've just hit the jackpot... so much of this was and is about shame". She described being criticised as a child, never being able to fulfil her parents expectations. After a while she started to feel unworthy, as though there was something intrinsically wrong with her. And of course this feeling of being defective or wrong is experienced in the current over-eating itself. Another client spent six months talking about her bereavements before she was able to gain enough trust to speak about her weight. This issue felt so painful to her and again was very bound up with her being unacceptable. She assumed that if she spoke about it I would reject her in some way. To open up to our shame both to ourselves and even more to others requires a lot of courage and considerable trust. Being over-weight only compounds the sense of shame for shame prone clients. Almost like a verification, an external badge of shame. "You said I was not good enough, well now I'm not! Being seen though is complex and other clients have said that being over-weight enables them to hide their sexuality. For these clients when they lose weight they can feel very vulnerable and a sense of shame because they start to feel more visible as they become thinner. It is as though their sexuality is more on display. We will discuss this later in the chapter on Recovery.

How Shame is Expressed

Shame is primarily expressed through the face. The person may hang their head and avert their gaze. There may be blushing or sweating. They may stare in a fixed manner their face looking frozen. The primary feeling is often of exposure and self-consciousness this may be experienced as shyness or embarrassment. The person may have thoughts that they are a fraud, they do not believe in themselves. They have thoughts of worthlessness and experience their body image as deficient. There is often a strong sense that they are unlovable or generally deficient. There can be a sense of emptiness.

Because shame is such a powerful and disabling emotion it often results in us adopting a personna or mask to desperately try to hide or deny the feeling. It is therefore not unusual if you experience shame in the company of other people that it is expressed as something else. People experiencing shame can therefore often appear contemptuous of others or angry , even rageful. They can transfer blame onto others or use sarcasm as a defence. This behaviour is often a projection onto others of the emotions they feel for themselves ie it is often safer to say "He's a load of rubbish!" than to acknowledge that I feel like rubbish!

Shame

Throughout the experiencing and expression of shame there will be a lot of muscular tension , a diminution of breathing and a sense of emotionally holding in the feeling. Shame is a very powerful emotion usually based upon profound pain. The natural expression would be to cry, howl or shout yet as this is usually seen as unacceptable in most situations the person will be required to try to hold all these feelings inside.

Defending Against Shame

As described above there are a number of ways in which we can block out our experience of shame.

Contempt

A client came to me who was very unhappy yet every intervention I made she challenged. She had a rather haughty, cool demeanour. I was aware in working with her that I quickly started to feel worthless as though I could not possibly say or do anything helpful. As I worked with her she slowly opened up and softened. It became quite apparent that she felt a powerful sense of shame and worthlessness. The feelings I experienced were primarily projections from her. Pushing the worthlessness onto me was less painful than facing these feelings within herself.

Exercise 7.1 Contempt & Shame

Think of someone who you feel contemptuous about. Write down the qualities which you feel describe this person: for example, aggressive, humourless, arrogant etc. Now apply these words to yourself in the form of a question:"Am I ever......humourless? Am I ever aggressive?"

Shame

Most human beings are a mixture of good and not-so-good, light and dark. Acknowledging our darker side enables us to stop projecting these qualities onto other people and denying our own authentic feelings

Envy

Another way to avoid shame is to be envious of others. We can focus on the perceived strengths of others both wanting and despising them at the same time. By giving other people strength or power we can disable our own sense of value or agency.

Exercise 7.2 Envy

Think of someone for whom you feel envy . Consider what are the qualities which you envy. Write down these qualities, whether you approve or disapprove, and again apply them to yourself.

Anger & Irritability

If we are angry and irritable with the world and other people this can be a great way to defend against allowing ourselves to feel the helplessness of shame. Anger can give us a sense of power. A client who had moved to a very disorganised and low morale department came to see me feeling very angry. Underneath she was ashamed that she felt she was letting down her clients because of the lack of support she was getting to do her job. Rather than acknowledge her sense of shame it was easier to project this out as anger onto her colleagues and onto me!

Shame

Exercise 7.3 Anger & Shame

Next time you feel angry with someone check what is happening underneath your anger. What are you upset or hurt about? Acknowledging the hurt or pain under the anger is the first step to resolving it! Sometimes the hurt is not related to the current issue but is more to do with an underlying sense of shame.

Often anger is like the froth on the top of a cappuccino. Underneath the froth is the hurt which has caused the anger. If we want to resolve our anger we need to understand the hurt.

Sometimes the hurt is not about something specific but is rather related to shame. We become angry because actually someone has said or done something which shames us. I recently went for a medical procedure which was uncomfortable. When I wriggled on the operating table the consultant in an exasperated tone said "Whatever is the matter!? This will go a lot better for both of us if you keep still". I went home and raged to my partner

"These bloody medics think they are gods! He should try having a catheter stuck in his groin whilst laying naked in a freezing cold operating theatre!"

When I had calmed down and decided perhaps his intervention although clumsy did not merit litigation I realised that actually it was about my own shame. As I man I felt I should be able to cope with some discomfort whereas in my mind he had shamed me in front of his team as someone who was worthless and deficient because he could not cope with some mild discomfort! Actually, he hadn't said I was worthless, I had.

Shame

So, our anger can mask our deeper experience of shame. Once I had realised the connection with shame my anger disappeared and I was left more with just the need to support myself in my experience.

Depression

A final way of responding to the experience of shame is to collapse in to depression. Rather than facing the expressions of shame, the sense of worthlessness, feeling like a fraud etc the person feels hopeless. They often have a sense that they can never succeed. They may feel inadequate in the face of other people's success.

Exercise 7.4: Shame Questionnaire

Read the shame questionnaire on the next page. If you tick more than 3 or 4 boxes this could indicate that you are quite shame-based and that the route out of your depression would be to work on your shame issues, which we will describe later in the chapter.

Shame

Shame Questionnaire

1. Do you avoid eye contact all or some of the time?
2. Do you blush easily?
3. Do you get over-heated or sweat easily?
4. Do you sometimes feel yourself freeze or feel like a rabbit caught in the headlights?
5. Do you feel exposed or vulnerable regularly?
6. Do you experience yourself as shy or self-conscious regularly?
7. Do you think that you are a fraud sometimes or all the time?
8. Do you have low self-esteem?
9. Do you have a negative body image?
10. Do you believe you are worthless or unlovable all or some of the time?
11. Do you feel empty all or some of the time?
12. When you are with other people do you sometimes adopt a contemptuous manner?
13. When you are with other people do you feel you should be perfect?
14. When you are with other people do you blame them if things go wrong?

Shame

15. When you are with other people do you become withdrawn?

16. When you are with other people can you be sarcastic?

17. When you are with other people are you self-deprecatory?

18. Do you experience envy of others?

19. Do you experience anger or rage which may cover your own sense of inadequacy?

20. Do you feel hopeless or that your life will never be successful?

Functional Shame

Shame can be a necessary corrective to behaviour, such as when a child reflects on stealing something, knows this is wrong, feels shame and returns the item. If we catch a domestic dog stealing food it appears to feel shame. It will hang it's head, avoid eye contact and if it could blush it probably would! These are forms of functional shame which regulate behaviour between us. The toxic shame we are describing arises not from teaching right and wrong but rather from a process of emotional rejection. How does this happen?

How Shame Arises

We have described earlier how needs occur through the awareness of sensation, the naming of the sensation, the possible experience of an emotion or an image and finally the expression of the need. This is a natural cycle which happens in all human beings. Shame arises when this process is interrupted by the family environment. Let's think how this happens. You have connected with your need you express it to your parents in the form of energy or excitement: " I want to get a bike!"and it is met with a negative response. This need, energy ,enthusiasm can be meet by a number of reactions:

- It is not accepted
- It is ignored
- It is rejected
- You are told you are bad for doing it
- You are withdrawn from or abandoned
- Your parent seems unavailable because they are overloaded, ill or injured physically or emotionally
- You are verbally or physically attacked

Exercise 7.5 How Shame Arises

Remember how your expressions of enthusiasm, energy or need as a child were met by your parents. Draw a map of the cycle of what typically happened , this would include:

- How you felt
- How you tended to express yourself
- The reaction of your Mum & Dad
- The reaction of your siblings
- Your response to their reaction
- Where this left you

Shame

Example:

    1. Excitement thinking about a new bike

    2. Speak quickly - trying to convince parents

    4. Feel deflated, angry. Less willing to express feelings again

    3. Met with boredom, lack of interest & iritability

When you have completed your map consider what would have really supported you.

If you are rejected now and then in a generally loving environment that is ok but if you are repeatedly met with the reactions above of being ignored or disapproved of this starts to become linked to you as a person.ie this is not being rejected because there is a problem with the specific request ie "I want a bike" this is being rejected because there is something wrong with me.

Jenny Mackewn describes this process as a "shame-bind": the shame becomes linked to the expression of the need. You learn that it's not ok for you to express your needs; yet because we all have needs therefore it is not ok for you to be you.

See the diagram on the next page

Shame

Shame Binds

Expressed Need

⬇

Rejection/ Disapproval/ Attack

⬇

Need Seen as Unacceptable

This cycle is repeated until:

⬇

Shame Bind

"My needs are unacceptable

Therefore I am unacceptable"

Collapse of Internal Support

⬇

Expression of Needs becomes Minimised or even Rejected

Sense of Self Shrinks

Shame-Based Personality is Created

Where the family environment does not provide interest, empathy and support you can see how the individual starts to operate from a place of shame. Their needs become minimised or even rejected, as in, "I should be strong" or " Don't wash your dirty linen in public". Sally grew up in

Shame

a family like this. When I first met her she had only come because her life and health were collapsing. Her first words were "I'm usually a strong person". Someone who is shame based may find it hard to acknowledge their needs. They have often been systematically trained over years to suppress and deny their needs:

Needs = "Bad"

The consequence of this is that needs become disowned and the individual is genuinely not really aware of their most basic needs. The need has lost its voice. Clients often will express a deep disconnection from fundamental and biologic needs such as being too cold, over-tired, thirsty, needing to pee, never mind needing affection or needing to talk. Recovery from shame requires an intense re-education in knowing your body, its sensations and needs!

The Internalising of Shame

The voice of the rejecting parent will become internalised as a portion of the self which attacks the self-that-has-needs. The child's internal world will become split into the persecutor ,"What's wrong with you?" and the victim "But I'm tired!"

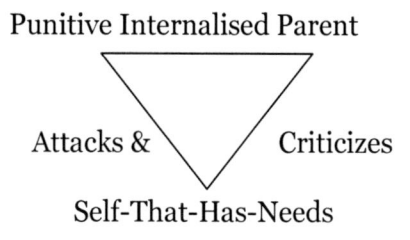

Punitive Internalised Parent

Attacks &   Criticizes

Self-That-Has-Needs

Shame

Fundamentally, because their needs were not acknowledged or met the child feels themselves to be unlovable. This is played out in the adult individual's inner mental life. They continue to re-cycle the rejection experienced as a child. There is a hostility towards themselves that may manifest in the punitive background commentary that runs alongside their daily life. "Oh there you go again!".There is an absence of Internal Support ie the ability to offer compassion and kindness towards the self because this has never been modelled to them.

All of this mean that it is also very difficult for shame-based individuals to get any External Support. To ask for support from others would be to acknowledge need and that is clearly not acceptable. My client who took six months to talk about her weight issues found it so difficult precisely because of her sense of shame not only about being over-weight but because she needed help and support itself.

The internal shaming process is known primarily as an experience of the body and face; it is not verbal, it is experiential not conceptual. It may take the form of squirming, (Yontef 1996), heat, tension, discomfort, a desire to hide or disappear, an explosion of defensive anger. It may include negative rules but is mainly known through being physically experienced.

Once the shame-bind has been created any expression of need which inadvertently is revealed to the person or others will trigger a sense of shame. Simply walking into a store to buy something may create shame , because it reveals need it creates a sense of shame. Asking for directions or to borrow sugar from a neighbour all of these simple everyday actions can trigger a sense of shame.

Shame

Exercise 7.6

Consider your own family and identify what was unacceptable to want or to express in your family of origin? Were your distinct needs acknowledged or ignored? This is not to suggest that your every need should have been met but rather that your expressed needs were met with some interest and understanding.

Recovering From Shame

Recognise that shame is an issue for you

Any change process begins with the recognition of a problem. Having read through this chapter decide if all or some of this applies to you.

Become aware of your body and its signals

Spend a little time each day actively trying to listen or catch the information from your body. Notice muscular tightening or tension in your body. Be aware of any mental images or emotions that go with these sensation. Try to adopt an attitude of curiosity towards your own body. "Oh, what is my body saying now?" As you become more aware of these signals try to incorporate this process into your decision – making. "Ok, my head says go on working, what does my body say?" Notice how you may push away the information from your body "Oh, I'm just being stupid". Validate your own experience – if **you** feel cold you are cold!

Shame

Start to become more fully expressive of needs.

As you become more aware of your sensations, images and emotions you will become more aware of your own needs. The next step is to allow yourself to be expressive of your needs. So, if you are cold you may need to express this and to ask if you can turn up the heating. Doing this will make you more visible and will reveal you have needs. This is precisely when you may experience a sense of shame. If needs are not acceptable by asking to turn up the heat you are potentially showing that you are not acceptable!!

So, to counter this you need to develop the internal mantra:

"It is fine for me to have needs

and to express them!"

I have put this in a "shameless" font size because this belief needs to be strongly and shamelessly held!! To recover from shame requires that we stop hiding, that we step in the spotlight and say "This is me , needs and all.... and I am fine!" The critical voice that will inevitably pop-up will need to be challenged repeatedly until you can start to live in the freedom of the mantra above.

Deal with the original scenes of rejection

I would encourage my clients attending for psychotherapy to imagine addressing the parent who had rejected their original needs. This "standing up" to the early source of neglect often seems to be very helpful. Expressing their sense of hurt and anger and stating that they are no longer willing to go on living the half life which the denial of needs creates can be very therapeutic.

Shame

Exercise 7.7 Recovering from Shame

If you wish to move forward from your sense of shame you will need to articulate your hurt and anger to your parents. This could be done as a conversation you have in your mind with them, or imagining sitting opposite your parent and literally telling them what their denial of your needs felt like. Alternatively, you could write all of this down in the form of a letter to them. I do not recommend that you actually speak to your parents. Moving on from your shame is something which needs to happen inside of you and anyway your parents may well react defensively and this will only compound your difficulty.

You may well experience a desire to protect your parents from your own anger or criticism. As stated before it is important to remember that you are criticising an element of their behaviour this does not mean that you cannot appreciate or love other aspects of them.

Development of an Internalised Positive Voice

In contrast to rejecting their rejection and the damage it may have caused you is the development of a positive internalised voice. Developing a friendly and compassionate internal voice is most important if you feel a sense of shame.

Exercise 7.8: The Internalised Positive Voice

If you can remember someone positive in your past, a grandparent, an aunt or uncle , a teacher try imagining what they would say to you about any given situation. If you are experiencing shame regarding something think, "What woud grandma have said?" Hopefully she would have encouraged and supported you. It is precisely this kind and

Shame

compassionate internal voice that will enable you to start to develop and grow again. To know that you are lovable is the final goal and this requires a kindly internal voice.

Visible – Invisible

Clients who experience shame often describe moving between the polarities of either feeling invisible, as though they do not exist, or overly visible where they almost feel as though people can read their minds or see their thoughts and feeling. If your needs were minimised or ignored as a child it is not surprising if you at times feel invisible. Equally, if your needs were seen as unacceptable it is not surprising if, when you feel your needs are seen, that **you** suddenly feel unacceptable.

Exercise 7.9: Protection

Try imagining a protective shield around yourself like the force field around a spaceship to keep out the incoming missiles, or picture a defensive aura around you or a screen or shield that protects your heart. Other people cannot see into us so it is important if you feel "seen into" that you develop an image to protect you. You could picture your chest having a smoked glass screen that appears if you feel too visible – so you can see out but that your heart is protected from an unwanted gaze. Imagine strong sliding doors that close over your heart if you feel invaded in some way. When you feel comfortable again you can open the doors.

Shame

The Management of Shame

Recovering from shame requires not only the re-building of your sense of self-love but also the ability to manage your experience of shame itself. Feeling shamed can in itself perpetuate the underlying sense of shame. So, if you start to feel yourself reacting from your sense of shame it is important to:

1. Start to breathe fully and deeply

2. Remind yourself it is fine to have needs and to express them

3. Remember that it is fine to be visible AND that your internal reactions are not visible to other people even if it feels like they are.

4. Remind yourself you have as much right to be here.

5. Imagine what your positive person would say

6. Remember you are lovable whatever happens

7. If you are a parent imagine what you would say to your child if they felt ashamed.

Copy the above onto an index card, carry it with you and consult it if you regularly feel shamed.

Shame re being Over-weight and Over-eating

A client who was over-weight described walking out of work one day eating an apple and another day eating a bar of chocolate. She was aware that eating the apple was ok but that when she ate the chocolate she imagined people saying "Fat cow... look at her stuffing herself even when she's walking down the street". Another client described going to a summer party where friends encouraged her to get up and dance and sing. She said she couldn't sing although she has a good voice and that she couldn't dance because she had a bad back which was not true. What she really felt was that she was terrified of being seen and being mocked because of her weight. Again, she experienced shame regarding herself even though these were friends who she knew liked and approved of her.

This highlights a very tricky issue regarding shame and weight. On the one hand it is crucial as this book has emphasised that we develop unconditional love and approval for ourselves yet if we dislike how we look because of the weight issues we need to approach any sort of change regime with compassion and kindness. Most people who over-eat have spent years attacking themselves and a central element of the change process is to begin to develop a less critical and kinder internal voice.

Summary

In this chapter we have explored

- Defining shame: Regarding oneself as disgusting, repugnant to others, loathsome, untouchable, unwanted, a bother or nuisance, not a gift.

- How shame is expressed: Shame is primarily expressed through the face. The person may hang their head and avert their gaze. There may be blushing, heat or sweating. They may stare in a fixed manner their face looking frozen. They may feel they are a fraud, incompetent, weak and as though they do not belong.

Shame

- Defending against shame via contempt, anger, envy, depression

- The shame questionnaire

- How shame arises through the negation of the child's needs. Not only do needs become seen as bad but the person experiencing the need develops a sense of being bad or wrong.

- Internalising shame: the critical parental voice becomes internalised as the primary voice within the mind of the child and then adult.

- Recovery from shame via body awareness, expression of needs, dealing with the original rejection, internalising a positive voice, moving from invisible to visible

- Managing shame incidents via breathing, the affirmation of needs, the expression of needs and the use of positive self-talk.

Chapter 8

Food, Eating & The Development of Identity

"I am utterly amazed at how closely my ways of dealing with problems, with reading matter, with movies, etc parallel my ways of dealing with food" **Gestalt Therapy Perls 1951:197**

The developing foetus in the womb is in a safe cocoon that is utterly merged physically and psychically with its mother. When the baby emerges into the world its initial food is the liquid milk from the breast of the mother. At this stage the baby sucks and draws the liquid into itself so there is still a minimal boundary between itself and the mother. Mother and baby have powerful biologic need of one another. The baby's identity both in the womb and in the early stages is therefore still very merged with that of the mother.

As the baby develops so it starts to be presented with increasingly solid food. At this stage the baby learns to start to bite and chew. If you have had several children you may have noticed how differently they deal with food. Right from the beginning some children will suck greedily on the nipple or bottle whilst others are less demanding. With solids they similarly adopt various behaviours towards their food. Chewing in a concentrated fashion or becoming dreamy and vacant as they chew.

Food, Eating & The Development of Identity

Exercise 8.1: How You Eat!

Sit down and eat some food in your normal way . As you eat be aware of how you feel. Notice the style in which you "attack" your food. Do you tend to eat quickly or slowly? Do you swallow some of your food whole or do you "liquefy" your food with lots of chewing? Do you focus directly on the food or do you sit and dream? Do you need to be distracted by the TV or by reading a paper or a book?

In his fascinating book **Gestalt Therapy** Fritz Perls describes how the process of eating parallels very precisely the developing identity of the child and in particular how the child absorbs the rules of its parents. For Perls the process of chewing is closely associated with the idea of "chewing over" information. He regarded chewing and masticating as an aggressive process of assimilating the food into the child's system.

Where children have been subject to a dominant style of parenting Perls believed that this was similar to being force-fed. The child has been effectively dominated or manipulated into the acceptance of various rules or ideas held by the parents. Noticing how you eat, as in the exercise above, will often reveal how you approach life and how you adapted to your parents style of parenting.

For example I will naturally eat quite rapidly and anxiously – I have to get the food in quickly and do not chew very much. This parallels precisely how I would live if I did not bring awareness to my style. I tend to rush at life with an anxious enthusiasm, bite off big chunks and then suffer the "indigestion" of being too quick. I do not always chew things over and will tend to believe what I'm told and swallow things down. Over time my style has really changed as I try to bring greater mindfulness to what I do. If I'm tired or low though I will probably tend to slip back into my default style.

Food, Eating & The Development of Identity

Exercise 8.2: Eating Mindfully

Prepare some food that you like you like. Sit for a moment and observe the colours, textures and aromas of the food.

Take your first mouthful and concentrate on the experience in your mouth. Eat slowly and mindfully. Chew deliberately until the food is well broken down. Allow yourself to experience fully the first mouthful of food before moving to the second. Be aware of any impatience as you pursue this exercise. If you become frustrated lay down your eating utensils, take a few deep breaths and then proceed to the next mouthful. Do not distract yourself with external stimuli. If you have a quick or impatient eating style you may find this exercise difficult or even quite challenging. This may be especially so if you are used to diverting yourself with external stimuli like a book or the TV.

Allowing yourself to eat slowly and mindfully will enable you to re-connect both with your food and also your body's experiencing of the food. If you wish to understand your habit of over-eating, developing a deeper understanding of your food consumption pattern will really help you change. Facing how you approach food though is no necessarily easy!!

In Fritz Perls book he notices how people who are "neurotic", want to avoid the "aggression" of chewing their food. ForPerls chewing was symbolic of our capacity to chew ideas. Being able to become a separate person with separate ideas is a central aspect for Perls of becoming a fully functioning adult. For Perls breaking down the food by chewing was similar to considering rules and information and deciding if they are valid or appropriate for you. What is apparent in working with many clients who over-eat is that they have always struggled with becoming fully distinct individuals as Perls describes. They have often been raised in a way which states or implies that they should simply accept what they are told – there should certainly be no discussion or argument regarding these issues.

This difficulty parallels the concepts of confluence or merger ie the child is often overly dominated by the parent and given the impossible paradox of "be yourself OR be loved". It is not surprising if most children chose to be loved but give up on becoming most fully themselves. Central to this difficulty is the avoidance of conflict. Clients who over-eat frequently report that they will do anything to avoid conflict and arguments. Yet if I wish to be fully myself it is inevitable that I will experience some "friction" in the world. Other people will not necessarily agree with my version of life. If I avoid conflict I will probably avoid being who I am!!

Example

As a child Jane was constantly criticised and compared unfavourably to her sister. Her mother would insist that she ateand "enjoyed" large family meals. If she was not hungry her mother would see this as a rejection of her food and of her as a person. At the same time Jane was criticised for being over-weight as a child. When she came to see me she would eat quite normally at home with her husband but then binge-eat secretly away from the family house. On her own she would eat rapidly and guiltily. Never feeling sufficiently loved even though she had "a good husband" – the secret food was her way of trying to gain the love and approval she sought. Of course the food was only ever a very temporary relief and was associated with a lot of shame and guilt regarding her behaviour.

Exercise 8.3 Needs & Difference

Start to become aware of your needs and the points where you have different needs to other people. Experiment with stating your different needs. This does not necessarily mean your need will get met but try becoming more used to the expression of the need in the face of disagreement. Very often if we were children of dominant/confluent parents we would expect a catastrophic outcome to disagreeing with our parents. This sets a pattern which we need to break. It is reasonable that we have different needs and that other adults may not like this but they need to accept our right to be different. If you catch yourself expecting a catastrophic outcome you need to challenge this view with a mantra such as "It's fine for me to be different" also "It's fine for you to disagree with me but not to abuse, belittle or patronise me because of the difference".

If you change your expectation of how your expression of needs will be met you will change your experience of what happens. If you normalise the expression of your needs and stop associating them with conflict, shame or being somehow unusual you will be met with a different response. As Ceser Millan demonstrates repeatedly on his TV show *The Dog Whisperer* the expectations of the dog owner determines to a large degree how the dog will behave!! If you expect conflict that is what you will experience. It is true that if for many years you have not expressed your needs people in your circle may initially find this strange or even difficult. However, if you stick to this new assertion it is remarkable how quickly these difficulties can be changed. If what you demand ie the right to express your need is reasonable most people will accept this,. Where they do not then you may need to consider whether these are people you want to be in relationship with.

Food, Eating & The Development of Identity

Where these people are relations and you wish to maintain the relationship you may need to reconsider the amount of contact which you are going to have with them. Remember, this not about you becoming a selfish person rather it is about you asserting your right to have and express your own needs. This is not an unreasonable request.

The Meaning of Food

Food you might say is just food and yet it seems as though because of the significant role it plays in our early life it often becomes something else. Given the importance of food in the life of the child food can be used by both parent and child as a way of asserting control or dominance. The child trying to dominate the parent may refuse food. The parent trying to control the child may make affection dependent upon the eating of food. As in the example above Jane's mother would suggest that if you reject my food you reject me! For Jane eating food away from her family was a source of comfort – she could feel safe from attack or criticism on her own and eat until she temporarily felt some inner relief.

Food therefore often becomes a source of substitute love. The sweetness or carbohydrate loading mimicking the warmth of affection. For those few minutes or even seconds before the self-attack kicks in we can feel whole again. Paul Mclean (1990) has suggested that substance abuse may be driven by the search for the appropriate brain chemicals which mimic the sense of love and affection. In the same way certain foods may help replicate this need for love. For Jane, to go and eat secretly away from her family certainly had the quality of an "affair" .To be driven to this may be precisely because Jane was seeking the bio-chemical" fix " that enabled her to feel temporarily loved.

Food, Eating & The Development of Identity

Exercise 8.4 Food & Control

Reflect upon the role that food played in your family life as a child? Were there issues of dominance or control expressed through food. What does food currently mean to you? Is food a substitute for something else in your life?

Summary

In this chapter we have explored and experimented with the following issues:

- In early development the identity of the foetus and mother are physically and psychically merged

- The young baby starts eating liquids initially progressing to solids it learns to chew and starts to assert its separate identity.

- Fritz Perls notices the difference between chewing food and swallowing whole. For him this symbolises our ability to "chew over" ideas and assimilate them rather than more passively simply accepting the rules and information we are given by our parents.

- Experiment and understand your eating style and how this reflects your approach to people and life in general

- To be fully functioning adults we need to be capable of understanding our needs and expressing them. We need to be able to discriminate between these needs and the ideas and needs of others, such as our parents. Conflict is an inevitable part of this process. If we avoid the conflict we will not be able to fully be ourselves.

Food, Eating & The Development of Identity

- Experiment with understanding and asserting your needs especially in the face of disagreement or expressions of difference.

- Adjust your life accordingly if friends and relatives will not accept the expression of your reasonable needs. This is not about becoming selfish but rather building a life in which you can more freely develop your confidence to become your own person.

- All sorts of psychological issues get played out through and around food. Become aware of what food meant in your family and what food means to you currently.

Chapter 9

Mindfulness & Over-eating

So far in this book we have been exploring a mainly psychological approach to over-eating. We have looked at how the patterns of love and affection, or the lack of them have affected how we currently function. I regard these approaches as the foundation stone for helping to re-build your view of yourself in relation to over-eating. However, this approach can be greatly enhanced by using Mindfulness to support your endeavours.

Practitioners of Mindfulness report that they feel calmer and more focussed. They experience a heightened sense of the here-and-now and seem less emotionally burdened by the past. These are all qualities which can really help to support the programme we have been discussing so far. Having used meditation for many years mindfulness is one of the most accessible ways to learn meditation. It is especially useful as it is not aligned to any religious practice and is easily available to improve the function of your body, mind and spirit.

Mindfulness and Over-Eating

Mindfulness-Based Stress Reduction was created by an American, Jon Kabat-Zinn, and colleagues at the University of Massachusetts. This programme was developed from the ancient practice of mindfulness as an accessible way for patients with a variety of conditions to help manage their illness or difficulties. The full training involves teaching participants meditative techniques which they can then use to support themselves. Much of what follows is based closely upon the teachings of Kabat-Zinn.

The Here & Now

As you will have noticed in the preceding chapters over-eating frequently occurs because of our difficulty in dealing with or expressing emotions. In a sense when we cannot express ourselves emotionally in the present it is because we are caught up in the past. We are operating, to use a computer analogy again, from old software. One way to resolve this problem is to go back – look at the old software and create some new programmes. This is what we have been doing in the earlier part of the book. The other way to approach the problem is to improve and intensify our connection with the here-and-now. This is the approach of Mindfulness.

Most people spend a lot of time regretting the past or worrying and catastrophising about the future. With the Mindfulness approach you are encouraged to repeatedly bring your attention to the moment. It is very easy for us to simply operate from our "automatic pilot". Through habit we tend to live in the way in which we drive. That is, we can drive for miles without really noticing the road or the scenery because our "mind is elsewhere". Try using the following exercise with the ten zones to develop the power of Mindfulness.

Mindfulness and Over-Eating

Exercise 9.1: Body Zones Awareness

Follow the instructions below or download the mp3 tracks of all the mediations available at www.dialogueconnsultancy.com

Imagine dividing your body into 10 zones. We will now work through the ten zones. Try simply noticing and trying not to judge what we find.

1. Brow & crown of your head
2. Eyes & temples
3. Mouth & Jaw
4. Throat
5. Arms, shoulders & hands
6. Chest, heart & solar plexus
7. Belly
8. Pelvis & Genitals
9. Legs
10. Feet

Get into a comfortable position lying or sitting. Bring your attention to the crown of your head. Be aware of any sensations. Whatever you experience simply try to accept it. If you feel any pain or discomfort acknowledge it and try not to judge it. Simply observe the crown of your head. Maintaining this attitude move your attention down your head to your forehead or brow. Be aware of any tension or holding. We can often hold tension in this place. Now moving your attention around the head to your temples. Again, simply noticing what you find, be aware of any judgement or criticism. Now moving your attention to your eyes. Be aware of any dryness or watering in your eyes. Notice any discomfort or relaxation. If thoughts arise simply return to the exercise. Now moving your attention to your mouth. Be aware of any tightness or holding. Notice the inside of your mouth ,is there any dryness? Be aware of your tongue and the teeth in your mouth. Notice the saliva.

Now moving out to your jaw. Be aware of any tightness or holding. Simply observe what you find. Now moving your awareness to your neck and throat. Notice any feelings inside your throat. Any tightness in the adam's apple. Be aware of your swallowing reflex. And now moving your attention to this whole area of your neck and head. Noticing how your head is supported on your shoulders. Continue in this fashion through the other six zones simply noticing and carefully observing what you find. Try to simply accept whatever is present. If thoughts arise simply return to the exercise

Practice this exercise every day for the next fortnight. Do not expect to feel anything especially different. You may find it difficult to maintain your concentration or focus. You may feel bored with the exercise. You may keep drifting off into thinking. All these reactions are fine. The point of the exercise is to simply follow the instructions. Over time, with repetition, you will find that this will start to encourage you to:

- Focus on the here-and-now

- Not be distracted by your thinking but to focus on one thing

- Become aware of how easy it is to judge what you find
- Develop a less judgemental more acceptant attitude
- Become aware of where and how you hold tension in your body

All of the skills developed by the Body Zones Awareness exercise can be generally helpful to you in developing a more peaceful and focussed way of thinking. In relating to issues of self-criticism and shame it can help you to simply accept yourself where and how you are. In term of body image it can also help you to become more accepting of your body and its current shape. This is crucial if you want to break the cycle of self-criticism. Breaking the old habits of self-criticism can take time and I would urge you to simply repeat the exercise every day for the next fortnight.

Exercise 9.2: Eating Mindfully:

As our daily activity on the mp3 we are using mindful eating

Having experienced the Body Zones Awareness exercise we need to develop our Mindfulness awareness into our daily activities. Choose a daily activity such as eating, showering, cleaning your teeth, washing the dishes, standing in a queue. Apply the same slow, careful attention to these tasks. Again, become aware of all the separate processes in the activity. Allow yourself to fully experience each aspect. With eating notice the aromas, the tastes and the textures of the food. Notice your impulse to rush or how your mind wanders away from the task of simply eating.

Mindfulness and Over-Eating

Mindfulness is not about spending hours sitting on a cushion meditating although for some people it can be. Rather it is about developing meditative techniques which you can use in your everyday life. The most important of these is Mindful Breathing and an associated and supportive technique, The Full Mindful Breath. You can use Mindful Breathing to sit and meditate and also you can use The Full Mindful Breath to help support yourself in your daily activities. Firstly let us look at Mindful Breathing.

Exercise 9.3: Mindful Breathing

Follow the instructions below or use the mp3 track

1. Sit in a relaxed and comfortable posture. Whether you sit in a chair, kneel or use a meditation stool it is important that your spine should be straight and erect. Allow your shoulders to drop.

2. Close your eyes

3. Become aware of your body and the sensation of the contact of your body with the chair or floor. Notice how your body starts to settle as you sit. Bring the same awareness as with the Body Zones exercise. Practice simply noticing how your body is.

4. Notice the movement of your stomach rising and falling as you breathe.

5. Bring your attention now to the breath. Breathe in a completely natural way. Do not use any sort of breathing technique. Observe the breath as you inhale and then as you exhale. Simply watch the movement of the breath as it flows into and out of your body.

Mindfulness and Over-Eating

6. As you try to maintain your awareness on your breath thoughts will probably arise. You may find yourself suddenly a long way away from your breathing. When you do simply return your awareness to your breathing. Notice any judgements you may make of yourself for losing your focus. Again, try not to get caught in the judgemental thoughts. Simply return to the focus on your breath.

7. Again, as you focus on the breath you may become distracted by your thoughts. If it is helpful label your thought ie say to yourself "Oh there I go again, thinking about Jane!" ... and then return to your breath focus.

Initially try this meditation for 10 minutes every day. The practice of this meditation has a number of benefits:

- As you practice the meditation you may find it is frustrating because your mind wanders. This is quite usual when you start to meditate. It is often called "monkey mind" – our minds constantly leap from one thing to another. Try to accept that your mind does this jumping, notice any judgements you make and simply return to the breath focus. Over time you will start to experience a new sense of focus and calm. Do not take my word for it though. Make a commitment to practice the Mindful Breathing Meditation for a fortnight and see what your experience is!

- Catching the judgements you make about the meditation is similar to the self-judgements we all continuously make. Practicing letting go of the judgement and returning to the breath focus can help establish in you a much less judgemental attitude.

Mindfulness and Over-Eating

- Over-eating often occurs because of the negative self-judgements we make. Learning to become aware of and diminish this habit can be very helpful to creating a kinder and more compassionate inner world! All the time in Love Myself Slim our overall goal is to develop a sense of greater compassion and kindness towards ourselves. As we do this our authentic compassion for the world will naturally grow

- Labelling your thoughts can help you catalogue and therefore let go of your thinking. A bit like giving a computer file a name so you can save and close it, labelling thinking can help your brain to switch off and cease worrying about an issue. Once the thought is labelled our brains are more likely to relax and move into a calm acceptant state. "Oh there I go worrying about work again".... and then you can return to the focus on breathing.

    Also, over time you will discover that your mind tends to get busy around certain subjects. This may be because they need attention or simply that you are "going around" an issue in a fairly un-productive pattern. If you notice you keep going around certain thoughts it may mean you need to give these issues some proper attention away from meditation OR decide that you need to accept there is no more you can do about this issue for the present. In the latter case, when the issue arises, continue practising simply returning to the breath in your meditation. This will help your brain to let go of struggling with the issue and acknowledge that for the moment you need to practice acceptance.

- Focusing on our breath enables us to move out of the fantasy world of what happened yesterday or the fear of what may happen tomorrow. When we meditate

- on the breath we are alive in the best place. The Here-and-Now. Allow the breath and the Here-&-Now to become an anchor – a safe haven.

Exercise 9.4: The Full Mindful Breath

Using the meditation above can have many benefits as described. Sometimes though in daily life we need a quick powerful technique to help calm us. If we are very anxious or dealing with someone who is aggressive then we can use breathing in a slightly different way to support us in our day to day activities. The following technique can help to rapidly calm you and enable you to become more grounded.

1. Most people breathe in the upper part of their chest. When they become stressed or anxious they will inhibit their breathing even further. Less oxygen goes to their brain and the mind becomes cloudy and unclear.

2. To breathe fully we need to start the breath from the belly. Place one hand on your belly, the other on your chest. Breathe in through your nose and allow your belly to expand. You should feel your belly pushing against your hand as it rises. Alternatively place both hands where your ribs end. As you breath in feel your ribs rising and expanding.

3. Continue the breath slowly and smoothly up allowing your chest to expand, you should feel a gentle expansion under the hand on your chest.

4. When your lungs are comfortably full breathe out through your mouth. Gently contract your muscles in your belly to help expel the air. Imagine using

Mindfulness and Over-Eating

your belly as a bellows to gently but firmly squeeze out the air

5. Finally relax your belly to prepare for the next inhalation

Practice this breathing technique for 5 minutes per day for the next fortnight. When you practice periodically give yourself the simple verbal instruction "Just slow down". As you get used to breathing in this way start using it at times when you feel stressed, anxious or panicky. Remember to remind yourself to also "Just slow down".

The Full Mindful Breath has a number of benefits:

- When you breathe like this you are breathing in the fullest possible way ensuring that you get a lot more oxygen than usual. This will help you think more clearly.

- This breath will rapidly bring you out of the fantasy of what might happen into the actuality of the present. With the calmness the breath creates this will enable you to act in a more rational, less emotionally driven way. Most of the time our fantasies of things are far worse than the reality. Bringing yourself calmly into the present will enable you to manage whatever is in front of you in a much better way!

- Breathing fully gives you a greater connection with the whole of your body. When we are frightened we tend to tighten and contract making ourselves smaller. This is a primitive survival mechanism. Breathing fully helps us to expand and feel more assertive and confident. Breathing fully encourages a confident posture which in turn will flip your mind into a more confident mode.

- Low confidence dogs curl their tails under. If you hold the dog's tail up its confidence will rapidly start to return. So if you are feeling low in confidence imagine holding up your metaphorical tail!!

Exercise 9.5 Fantasy & Fact

Think about a time when you were quite unwell or someone close to you was quite unwell with a condition with which you were unfamiliar. When you first learnt of the diagnosis what imaginings went through your mind about what or how this illness might be and how it might effect you or them? Then consider the actual course of the illness. How accurate was your fantasy about the illness?

Or

Remember a place you loved as a child and then returned to as an adult. How was the memory of the place and then how did the reality compare?

In both cases there is the actuality of the illness or the place and then there is the interpretation or meaning we make of it. When I was diagnosed with a completely blocked major artery of my heart my initial reaction was that my whole life would fall apart and that I'd probably die! Whilst the reality was not altogether pleasant it was considerably more prosaic. I spent quite a lot of time lying on a sofa unable to do much and feeling rather sad and sorry for myself. The block was cleared and after a few false starts I returned to full health.

Equally, I could have assumed that because heart procedures are so routine it was a foregone conclusion that I would be fine and yet of course something like 5% of patients

Mindfulness and Over-Eating

undergoing angioplasty do not survive! Neither interpretation of events could be seen as very balanced.

Similarly, we can recall places with a gilded memory. I remember a huge tree in endless woods with a great bough that we young children used to happily bounce upon for hours. In my memory the sunshine dapples through the fresh green leaves of spring onto this special scene. Returning as an adult it was a scrappy little copse with a small tree and rubbish blowing about! Our view of reality is our interpretation:

"ACTUALITY" + INTERPRETATION

=

OUR VIEW OF THE WORLD

Thoughts are not Facts

Meditating can help us to see how we create our interpretations of the world. We do this through our observation of thinking. What do I mean? Over time as we observe our thoughts arising and disappearing in meditation we notice that our thoughts simply come and go. Thoughts are not as solid as we think! For example, Bill appears to treat us badly in a meeting. Bill behaves badly but what we often think and jump to, is that Bill is not a very nice man. Meditating after this meeting it may go around in your mind how Bill behaved and how you find him unpleasant. Later, we learn that Bill's mother died last week. Suddenly Bill is no longer a bad man but a man who behaved badly because he was grieving! We feel sympathy for him, no longer judge him and our initial interpretation of his behaviour is forgotten.

Mindfulness and Over-Eating

Learning to meditate and to try to drop our judgemental and interpreting mind can enable us to develop greater equanimity. We can never stop making interpretations but we can become more aware of how our thinking can rapidly lead us into the wrong conclusions about the world. As Jon Kabat Zinn succinctly puts it

"Thoughts are not facts"

As you continue to practice meditation you may discover the pure awareness which lies beneath or beyond thought. Even if only glimpsed initially momentarily this expanded state of consciousness can be of tremendous support in helping you develop a calmer and more compassionate sense of yourself.

Thinking and thought can be a wonderful tool but it can easily lead us, as I have demonstrated, into a false analysis of events. Where we have a history of being criticised and or of suppressing our own emotional response we can develop thinking habits which are not useful.

Exercise 9.6 Thinking Traps

Notice how many of the following thinking habits you get into over a day or week:

- Expecting perfection
- Catastrophising – expecting the worst
- Judging myself and or others harshly
- Highlighting and focusing on what I consider my weak areas

Mindfulness and Over-Eating

- Judging myself useless because of one thing whilst ignoring all the positives
- Thinking about things in a very rigid or black and white way
- Jumping to conclusions about people or events (as in the example above about Bill)
- Confusing thoughts with facts

I engage in most of these every day because it seems many of us do!! However, the trick is to try and catch yourself doing it and over time your automatic thinking patterns will have less power over you. Simply developing an awareness that you tend to catastrophise can then help you to limit this tendency: "Oh there I go again assuming the worst about the future... deep breath ... Try to trust the future can be good!"

Where you find yourself engaging in any of the above thinking patterns try adopting an attitude of kindly curiosity or bemusement! Be you at 80 years old looking back with kind consideration viewing this issue within the scope of a long and full life.:

"Is it really true you are completely useless because you did not get A* for your essay?"

Pleasant & Unpleasant Experiences

Catching the thinking patterns above can have a big impact upon how we construct the meaning of the next minute, hour, day, week month, year and life itself! Try the following exercise to notice how you create pleasant and unpleasant events.

Mindfulness and Over-Eating

Exercise 9.7: Pleasant & Unpleasant Experiences

1. Notice in the next week some pleasant things that happened to you. Be aware of the thoughts, feelings, images and body sensations in involved in this experience. Write down the event or experience and note your reactions.

2. Similarly, notice in the next week some unpleasant things that happened to you. Be aware of the thoughts, feelings, images and body sensations in involved in this experience. Write down the event or experience and note your reactions.

With the meditation you are encouraged to be less reactive to your thoughts ie when a thought arises you simply notice the thought and return to the focus of your breathing. In the same way you may notice with the pleasant and unpleasant events your body and mind tend to react to stimulus.

Occasionally we have jet aircraft fly over our house. I notice when I am meditating that even before a thought arises my body can tense up at the noise. I am reacting. The next step is that I will feel irritation. " Bloody jets spoiling my day!!" However, if I am aware of tensing I can pre-empt the irritation. I simply say "Ok, the wind has changed direction so we have jets coming over today. That's how it is!" **Instead of reacting I respond**. When I react I have no choice - when I respond I do have choice! This means that instead of fighting the inevitable and having "a bad meditation" I can enjoy my practice in the acceptance of the planes.

As Kabat Zinn notes, reacting to experience broadly falls into three categories:

Mindfulness and Over-Eating

1. **Aversion**: I want to stop the experience I am having or avoid an experience that is coming. I push away my here-and-now experience

2. **Indifference**: I go off somewhere mentally, this will often happen if we doing a "boring" routine activity like waiting in line at the check-out. Again I escape from the moment by moment experience.

3. **Attachment**: I try to hold onto the current experience or wish for some other experience which is not currently happening. I cling to the present, often fearful that it will not last. Alternatively, the present is never enough because I am overly attached to what I feel "should" be happening. I cling to the present or my fantasy of what it "should" be.

Again, practising Mindful Breathing can help to highlight how we tend to "go off" in our minds, push an experience away or cling to a pleasurable experience. Any of these reactions can prevent us simply staying with the focus of the breath in the moment. You may wonder how any of this helps you? Well, these are also all ways in which we can push away our emotional experience, cling to it or simply drift away from it in daily life.

If at the core of over-eating is our inability to acknowledge and express emotions then these are all ways in which we clearly prevent ourselves from expressing the full emotional range of who we are as human beings. To summarize then, be aware of how you react rather than respond to your day to day experiences. Notice how you can "catch" a reaction and choose rather to respond by using breathing, slowing down and then choosing a response. As Victor Frankl who survived the Nazi concentration camps says:

Mindfulness and Over-Eating

Between stimulus and response

There is a space

In that space lies our freedom and

power to choose our response.

In our response

Lies our growth and freedom

Exercise 9.8: Meditating on Your Body

Follow the meditation below or download and listen to the mp3

This meditation is a development of the Mindfulness of Breathing Meditation. Although we start with the focus on the breath we then expand our awareness to imagine breathing into our body. As you practice this meditation try to adopt a compassionate and kind attitude towards yourself. Your body is doing the best it can for you and it is the only body you have! Notice any criticisms or disparagements you may make and then return to the focus upon your breath. You can initially take 10 minutes with this meditation. Having learnt the two main meditations Meditation on Breathing and Meditating on The Body you can use either or both of these to regularly meditate with. The amount of time you take is up to you. Anything from 10 minutes to 45 minutes will be helpful for you.

1. Bring your attention to your natural breathing. As in the Mindful Breathing Meditation simply observe your breathing. When thoughts, feeling or sensations

arise simply notice them, label them, tell yourself it is fine think or feel whatever you are experiencing and return to the breath focus. Allow the breath to act as an anchor of stillness to help calm and centre you.

2. As you continue to breath simply observing the in-breath and the out- breath allow your awareness to extend to the whole of your body. One way to do this is to allow your mind's-eye to trace an imaginary line around your body shape. Now move the focus of your attention from the fine point of your breath

3. Expand right out to the edge of your body. Now visualise that you are not just breathing into your lungs but into the whole of your body.

4. If thoughts, feelings or sensations arise remind yourself it is fine to have thoughts and feelings, return to the focus of your breathing and then again try to expand your awareness out into your body.

5. Try to stay with this body awareness for the duration of your meditation whilst observing the arising and disappearance of thoughts and feelings

Micro-Meditation

As we noted earlier Mindfulness practice is not just about meditating for long periods it is about attempting to incorporate a certain "attitude of mind" into your daily life. If you can bring this awareness into your activities life will certainly start to improve. Using the Micro- Meditation is a way to ensure that you are remembering this attitude and that it is not just reserved for the ten minutes when you formally practice Mindful Breathing or Meditating on The Body. Once you have learnt the three stages, outlined below,

Mindfulness and Over-Eating

you can take as much time or as little to do this process. You can also use this meditation if you are troubled in your feelings and thoughts.

Very often when we become stressed or anxious we have lost good contact with ourselves. We are in a way off-balance and frequently no longer in the present moment. We have become pre-occupied by a thought, emotion or physical sensation. Often we have regressed to an earlier state, expecting something awful will happen or worried about what happened yesterday. We all continually flux between the here-and-now and these inner fantasy states. This is quite normal. However, when we become stressed we are usually becoming quite dis-engaged from ourselves and the present environment. You can regard the Micro Meditation as a way to rapidly re-connect with yourself.

Exercise 9.9: Micro-Meditation

Follow below or use the mp3 download track.

1. **Contact**: Say the following sentence "Here-and-now I am aware...." now check-in with your thinking, feeling, physical sensation and finally notice the environment you are in and what your response is to this. Describe to yourself what you find "Here-and-now I am aware I feel sad and that I am pre-occupied thinking about Ruth. I have a knot in my stomach. When I look out of the window I notice the sunlight falling on the flowers in the window box". Label what is happening overall "Oh, there I go again getting in a state about Ruth". If you feel you are quite stressed use 3- 5 Full Mindful Breaths ie breathing slowly and deeply from the belly to help calm yourself then return to breathing normally.

Mindfulness and Over-Eating

2. **Focus**: Bring your attention to your natural breathing. As in the Mindful Breathing Meditation simply observe your breathing. When thoughts, feeling or sensations arise simply notice them, label them, tell yourself it is fine think or feel whatever you are experiencing and return to the breath focus. Allow the breath to act as an anchor of stillness to help calm and centre you.

3. **Expansion**: As you continue to breath simply observing the in-breath and the out- breath allow your awareness to extend to the whole of your body. One way to do this is to allow your mind's-eye to trace an imaginary line around your body shape. Now move the focus of your attention from the fine point of your breath to expand right out to the edge of your body. Now visualise that you are not just breathing into your lungs but into the whole of your body. If thoughts, feelings or sensations arise remind yourself it is fine to have thoughts and feelings and return to the focus of your breathing. As you continue to breathe if you feel sufficiently relaxed you might even extend the imaginary line around your body out to incorporate the room you are in, the building, the city, the country, the planet, the universe. Remember though that the focus remains the breath and the body that if your mind starts to roam into pictures or thoughts then gently return to the breathing filling your whole body

Only ever take this as far as you personally feel comfortable. For many people imagining the space around them helps to develop both a sense of connection between them and their world and it helps give a sense of perspective. In this sense we are both connecting intensely with our environment and also ourselves. All of this is occurring in the Here-and-Now which can help you re-connect away from the stress you were previously experiencing.

When I use the Micro-Meditation I find it helps to jolt me out of whatever pre-occupation was bothering me and help support me back to a bigger sense of myself whilst reducing the scale of the thing that was troubling me. Again, do not take my word for it but rather experiment and see what you find!

This is a lot of words but can be done in two or three minutes. Sit at your PC or wherever you happen to be. Check in with your current state. Take a couple of deep breaths if necessary. Focus on your ordinary breathing and then expand your awareness out to incorporate your whole body. Think CFE if that helps:

Contact – Focus – Expansion

Barriers to Meditation

We can prevent ourselves from meditating in many ways:

- Just to give yourself the time may be an issue. Is it ok for me to sit down and stop for 10 minutes? Many people, especially women are programmed to be very busy and to never stop. They operate in what I call Doing Mode ie they are constantly doing things yet rarely change gear into Being Mode. Being Mode is about experiencing the moment. It does not have goals

- In the same vein we may be addicted to mastery and regard pleasure as something superficial and irrelevant ie we are constantly drawn to achievement

Mindfulness and Over-Eating

and the organisation of things rather than enjoying, for example, the pleasure of what we have mastered. Someone I knew spent hours organising a personal library so it was all carefully catalogued but then rarely spent time in this lovely book-lined room actually reading!

- We may question how stopping and sitting and breathing and focussing our attention can help anything, especially a weight problem! All l can say is that I would encourage you to try and find out for yourself what the benefits may be. What I would say though is, try to make a commitment to the exercises

- in this section for a month, practicing on a daily basis. Then decide whether it has merit for you.

- When we meditate we may feel that we are useless because our mind leap about and focus is impossible. This is utterly normal. Most people struggle. The trick is to try and let go of the criticism and just keep returning to the focus upon the breathing. Like any skill it takes a little time and it will come.

- Some thoughts or feelings can be very "sticky" – they keep coming back. Within the meditation I would encourage you to try to practice acceptance that this is currently where your mind is. Always return to the breath. Away from the meditation it may be there is work you need to do to get on top off this particular issue.

- Meditation is not a panacea. There may be some issues where you need professional help. If you keep getting stuck on certain issues you may need to seek counselling or some other form of help.

Mindfulness and Over-Eating

Much of the material in this chapter is based upon Jon Kabat Zinn's teaching on Mindfulness. Check the bibliography for his books which can offer much greater detail on this wonderful approach to meditation.

Summary

In this chapter we have explored:

- A definition of Mindfulness
- The importance of the Here & Now
- Body Zones Awareness
- Eating Mindfully
- Mindfulness day to day
- Mindful Breathing
- The Full Mindful Breath
- "Thoughts are not Facts"
- Thinking Traps
- Pleasant-Unpleasant Experiences
- Meditating on The Body
- Micro-Meditation
- Barriers To Meditation

Chapter 10

Compassion & Self-Esteem

At the heart of this book is the simple yet profound idea that compassion and kindness needs to be at the centre of who we are. A felt sense that we can love ourselves, not egotistically, but with a genuine respect and warmth for who we are. This is not for moral reasons, although it will clearly make for a better world, but because when we treat ourselves with genuine kindness we function more effectively and with greater balance and wisdom. If you want to change any pattern of abuse, including over-eating, it needs to start with transforming the way you feel towards yourself.

As Dr Paul Gilbert says in his book The Compassionate Mind:

"Focusing on kindness, both to ourselves, and to other people, stimulates areas of the brain and body in ways that are very conducive to health and well being. Researchers have also found that, from the day we are born to the day we

Self Esteem: Generating Compassion & Kindness

die, the kindness, support, encouragement and compassion of others has a huge impact on how our brains, bodies and general sense of well-being develop. ... So it turns out that kindness and compassion are indeed paths to happiness and well-being" Gilbert 2009:4

Working with an obese client recently we discussed how punitive and critical her mother had been. This had resulted in my client having a highly critical Internal Voice. She would chide and criticise herself all day long. At the end of one particular session I naively asked her how it would be to start to consider herself as "lovable". She looked at me as though I was from another planet!

On the next session she seemed confused and slightly angry. "I just do not get this lovable bit. I am not lovable, there is nothing lovable about me!". We spent the next half hour exploring what her friends think of her, what her colleagues say about her, what her family think of her, what her customers say about her. All these people would describe her as "kind, open, honest, loving"... they described "lovable" qualities. Confronted with this information it was almost as though my client felt cornered. "Yes, they may see me like that but I can't because I'd be .... big-headed then, wouldn't I?".

Children of critical parents not only tend to internalise the criticism they internalize the critic. They become their own worst critic. Crucially, this is usually under-pinned by another meta-rule which states that:

"It is not acceptable to feel positive and good about yourself... (often followed by) .... because this will make you full of yourself or big-headed!"

This is not only a classic family rule but sadly it is also often a major cultural norm. Certainly in the UK there is an

Self Esteem: Generating Compassion & Kindness

enormous culture of "Do not blow your own trumpet!. In some ways this is good because it makes for a more modest less aggressive attitude yet in my therapeutic experience it frequently becomes a way for clients to minimise their sense of self-worth. "I cannot feel good about myself because people won't like it i.e me like that". Ironically, being "full of self" rather than being seen as a negative could be a definition for how it is to feel happy... ie in a state of happiness people often describe feeling "full".

Exercise 10.1: Generating Love

Sit down somewhere quiet. Visualise a person or animal whom you unconditionally love. Consider them for a few minutes. Become aware of the feeling in your body as you do this. Notice the smile on your face or the warmth in your heart. Now, mentally remove the person you were thinking of and replace them with yourself!

Be aware of what happens in your body as you contemplate yourself. Notice any changes in your bodily reaction. Is your smile as broad ? Is your heart as warm? If there is a reduction in your bodily reaction when observing yourself give yourself time to think about this. How come you are not as deserving of love as your friend or your dog?

Go back to visualising the first person or animal. Allow the feeling of love to generate and then think of yourself again. This time try to actively offer this love to yourself. Try to drop your demand for perfection and be more accepting as you would with the first person or animal you thought of. If this is a difficult exercise for you keep repeating it trying to develop a compassionate and kind attitude towards yourself.

Self Esteem: Generating Compassion & Kindness

Knowing who we are and that we have various attributes and skills that all come together in the unique package of who we are seems wise. Respecting and valuing our own attributes and skills seems healthy. Without this inner sense of value there is no anchor and then we will simply be blown around by the latest opinion or valuation we pick up on from other people. Generating a realistic and healthy sense of our value is central to our mental health.

Some religions promote the idea of negating ego, always putting other people first or having no personal needs. My view is that we can only negate ego if we have one! What I mean is that you can only develop a sense of genuine spirituality if you have acknowledged both your weaknesses AND your strengths. If you essentially do not feel good about yourself trying to negate your ego or developing a sort of false piety is likely to make you feel worse. Knowing your strengths and value is healthy. Of course, bragging about them is tedious and boorish and probably would indicate that they are not qualities which you are really secure about!

Exercise 10.2: The Inner Mounting Flame

Consider all the positive people in all the facets of your life, family, work, social life etc. What would they say about what they value about you as a person? Imagine sitting all these people around you in a circle. Go around the circle and let each person say a few words about you.

Allow yourself to breathe deeply and slowly as you draw these compliments down into your heart. Now picture a small flame inside your heart. Each time someone says something kind or positive imagine the flame gets a little stronger. Finally, when everyone has spoken you can say a

Self Esteem: Generating Compassion & Kindness

few words about what you value, like, love or respect about yourself.

Now sit quietly and simply picture the flame. However small it is remember you are now the keeper of your own flame. In the past maybe other people really influenced that flame. Maybe attacking or diminishing the flame. Now you have the choice and the chance to nurture your own flame. Do this by periodically repeating this exercise. If you have had years of self-criticism it may seem strange to be offering yourself kindness and love. You may feel awkward, uncomfortable or foolish. Simply note these responses and return to offering yourself affirmation, kindness and compassion.

Life constantly throws up challenges which can apparently attack our sense of self-esteem. Our sense of value needs to not be totally "field-dependent". What I mean is that whilst I need to listen to the feedback from the world I need to not be unduly influenced by it ie dependent upon the world for my sense of value.

Exercise 10.3: Depth Acceptance

Sit down somewhere quietly. Take a few Full Mindful Breaths. Say to yourself:

" I chose to be here today and I choose to like and love myself exactly how I am. I love and cherish myself as I am today". Picture the flame in your heart and imagine it burning strongly and brightly" If doubts or uncertainty arise repeat the affirmation. Even if you cannot fully accept the statements try repeating them to see if they might become a way you could think. Your mind may counter with critical or hostile thoughts "But you're fat!" or "You look awful!" Irrespective of this chose to direct love towards yourself as you are! If you want to develop or grow including getting slimmer you need

Self Esteem: Generating Compassion & Kindness

to start with developing a greater compassion and kindness towards yourself. Compassion does not happen tomorrow it always begins right now with you where you are today!

If I simply react to the world I will constantly be pulled in different directions. Developing a strong inner sense of my value can really help me be more responsive and les reactive. At times of difficulty my internal flame may waver yet this is useful information as I may then move into my role as "keeper of the flame". If this occurs practice the meditations above, reflect upon your achievements to date and consider how those who love you value and respect you.

Self-Esteem & Anger or Rage

If you struggled with the two preceding exercises it maybe because of the anger or rage you feel towards those who inhibited your sense of value and self-esteem. This anger may be something you know about or something which is primarily out of your awareness.

As stated earlier in the chapter on suppressing anger we need to discriminate between our general feelings for our parents and feelings about particular ways in which they behaved. If we were criticised a lot or our needs were ridiculed or diminished we may well feel anger or even rage towards our parents or siblings.

Sally tried to love her mother yet hated the way she would always find fault with her behaviour. When Sally tried to feel warmth or compassion towards herself it frequently became blocked because she became angry that this care and affection had not come from her mother. Sally needed

Self Esteem: Generating Compassion & Kindness

to express her anger, let go of expecting affection from her mother and by so doing clear a space to enable her to start feeling some genuine kindness and compassion towards herself.

Sally achieved this over some months by reflection, talking and engaging with the following exercises. These exercises may take you days, weeks or months depending upon the intensity of your feeling and your desire to change:

Exercise 10.4: Expressing Hurt & Anger

Write a letter, which you are not going to send, expressing what you found difficult about your mother/father/siblings behaviour. If there is more than one person write them separate letters. Make sure the letter is fully detailed expressing the hurts and disappointments you experienced. If you have a confidante or counsellor, someone you can really trust read the letter out loud to them. This will help you externalise your feelings regarding these issues. Allow yourself to experience and express any emotions related to this fully.

In this stage you may wish to express some of your anger more physically by getting a punch bag and hitting it or using cushions to hit. Alternatively working out hard at the gym or exercising hard whilst reflecting on your anger. With all these expressions of anger ensure you take physical care of yourself and do not damage yourself. In this stage you need to be allowing the emotion whether of hurt, anger or disappointment to move from inside to outside so that it is no longer blocking your energetic system.

Self Esteem: Generating Compassion & Kindness

Exercise 10.5: The Kind Parent

After this at some point write a letter to yourself from the viewpoint of a kind and caring parent. " I know this was a difficult time for you etc". Reflect on what they (ie you) experienced as a child. Acknowledge the difficulties and then encourage them (ie you), to let go of demanding any further love.

"For years you have sought this affection or affirmation from your parents and they have been unable to give it. It is time to stop completely and utterly wishing for this. You must now let go of this demand and let go of the anger attached to it. You are the only person hurt by this anger and it changes nothing".

Many people spend years of their life in a state of fruitless yearning for love which cannot be given. Whilst it is deeply sad, in the end we have to accept that sometimes people are incapable of feeling or showing love because of the difficulties in their own parenting. Trying to manipulate, coerce, demand that we be loved on our terms will not work.

Exercise 10.6: Grieving The Love You Wanted

In the next stage you may well feel deep sadness or a sense of grieving that you are letting go of something very precious to you. What you are letting go of is your fantasy of the "good parent", the "good brother or sister". Most people hold an image of how their parents or siblings "should" be. Frequently, this does not accord with how these people really are. Although this period may be very painful you are moving out of fantasy into the actuality of how your life is. Although it is painful you will find that over time it becomes much easier to bear. We all have different ways of grieving. One way might be to take a photograph of the person. Express how you have felt let down by them. Allow yourself

Self Esteem: Generating Compassion & Kindness

to cry, try to let some of this feeling of loss move from inside to outside.

Exercise 10.7: Forgiveness & Acceptance

Having allowed yourself to grieve, reflect on your parents. If they were critical or could not give you love it was because of some failure of compassion in their lives. Sally explained how although she was always criticised her mother showed a lot of affection to her sister. This caused Sally considerable pain. No doubt something happened in Sally's mother's life which caused her to cut-off. Maybe she was criticised a lot and saw that as good parenting. Maybe she had a sibling who got more affection than her and so it was unconscious payback time! Sally was being punished for what her mother never had.

Rather than continuing to be angry it is time to offer understanding and forgiveness to your parents. To see them within a generational chain of your family. They could only parent as well as they were parented. Regard this as an opportunity to break this dysfunctional cycle and move forward.

Exercise 10.8: Clearing The Space for Love

Sit quietly. Imagine breathing in light and breathing out black smoke as a representation of all the hurt and pain. Clear a peaceful and bright space inside you. As you breathe out all the negativity and anger imagine as you breathe in that you are not only drawing in light but also love. Draw the love down into your heart as you continue to breathe in love and breathe out love. Imagine that you have transformed your inner landscape to one which is full of light and love.

Self Esteem: Generating Compassion & Kindness

By letting go of your "fantasy of love" you clear the space to start to be more compassionate and kind with yourself. You are no longer in a state of permanent deficit but can receive love from others and start to direct it towards yourself.

Exercise 10.9: Finding The Love You Need

Start to look for love, intimacy or communication elsewhere. As Sally said: "But if I give up hoping for love from her I will be lost. Who else can love like a mother?" And the answer, of course, is: "But you are lost anyway. You are yearning for something the other person cannot give. You have to let go and start to see the love that naturally surrounds you and will surround you more if you give up on this hopeless quest!"

Letting go of my fantasy of parental love delivered in the way in which I demanded was one of the most painful parts of my development. Yet equally it is highly liberating because you can then become your own person and you can start to look around at all the love, intimacy and communication which is available from friends and colleagues. Mostly when we are infatuated with love coming from one source we are utterly blind to that which surrounds us in our day-to-day life.

Ironically, when we give up demanding love from someone, that is the point when we may discover that although they cannot love us in the way we want, we may suddenly see other things which they offer, to which we were blind

Self Esteem: Generating Compassion & Kindness

Blocking Compliments: Staying in the Negative Bubble

To return to our theme of self esteem and compassion. Clearly, anger, rage, hurt and disappointment can block our emotional energy, These emotions leaves us in a space of negativity about ourselves and the world. This stops the flow of compassion and kindness which is so imperative for our mental well-being. The development of self-esteem and confidence is then, in turn, blocked.

Further, if we are used to not feeling good about ourselves we will typically block out any in-coming positive messages. We therefore perpetuate living in the past and block out the actuality of our present life. We remain in the negative bubble created in the past. This helps us to maintain the false belief that we are "useless". A bit like the military saying we have 'incoming fire' the emotional system is on alert to "incoming compliments" and responds accordingly. "Oh, that's fine!" "That's what we do!". Instead of acknowledging and taking in the compliment we bat it away. Doing this means we do not value ourselves or the other persons experience of us. We remain intent on maintaining our negative view of ourselves. Instead the next time someone compliments you think of the compliment as a being a beautiful smoothie!

Exercise 10.10: The Self Esteem Smoothie

So, imagine you have just been complimented. Consider the compliment like your favourite drink. Imagine sipping at the drink. Taste the sweet taste of the affirmation. As you breathe in imagine the liquid going down your throat. On the in-breath imagine drawing this nectar down into your body. How far can you allow this compliment to go? Do you

Self Esteem: Generating Compassion & Kindness

block it or can you allow yourself to draw it right down into your heart? Can you allow yourself to be touched by the fact that this other person saw you and valued you? However small the thing was it clearly affected them and enabled them to see you and appreciate you? From their perspective you are special! Can you allow yourself to be special just for this moment? If you find that you block, maybe at the throat or in the upper chest try to breathe deeply and slowly. Relax and try to allow the warmth of the compliment to penetrate a little deeper into your being.

Faced with someone giving us an actual compliment breathe deeply and slowly. Try to calm yourself in the face of the embarrassment, shyness or desire to run! Try to accept that the reality of the other person is that they are pleased with you. As they speak use the in-breath to draw the compliment down into your body. Try to allow the praise into your heart. When they have gone repeat the compliment a few times. Savour the affirmation. Maybe write it down if it helps you to hold it.

Storing Affirmations and Compliments

If we wish to develop greater self-esteem we not only need to become "open" to the affirmations in our present life we need to find a way to hold these positive messages. It is easy to dismiss and forget how you are regarded if you tend to block compliments and affirmation. A bit like reading your CV you can sometimes be surprised by what you have done and not altogether recognise yourself as the person on the CV. In this exercise you need to create a mental receptacle or "treasure chest" to hold all the good things about your life.

Self Esteem: Generating Compassion & Kindness

Exercise 10.11: The Self-Esteem Treasure Chest

Picture a box, a casket, an urn, a chest any receptacle which has meaning for you. Imagine this receptacle in your heart standing next to the flame. Remember something positive someone said. If you cannot access this take a compliment from me! Well done for getting this far in the book. If you have been doing all the exercises or even thinking about all these concepts you are doing well. You are beginning to make a difference in your own well-being. Take this compliment and imagine placing it in your receptacle. Now think about your life and all those people in your life who may have said positive things to you or about you. Place these compliments in the receptacle as well.

As a variation on this exercise you may want to actually write down things people have said to you on separate pieces of paper and place them in an actual container rather than one in your imagination. Either approach can be helpful. The important thing is that you stop dismissing compliments and affirmations and start to recognise how you are valued. If there is little current affirmation of you remember affirmations from the past and work towards changing your situation to create a more affirming environment. If you plant your flower in impoverished soil it may not flourish!

At times of difficulty return to your actual or visualised store of compliments. A bit like an old pile of photographs rummage through them and remember how you are loved!

Exercise 10.12: Feathers & Pillows

Another way to picture self-esteem is to think of every compliment or affirmation as a feather. In itself a feather is very light but if you fill a pillow case with feathers you create something which is beautifully soft yet very supportive

Self Esteem: Generating Compassion & Kindness

Exercise 10.13: Physical Self Esteem: Walk The Talk

Whilst it is important to generate a sense of value from using a cognitive or visual approach self esteem is also something which is manifested physically in your body. Think of the posture of someone who has good confidence and self-esteem. Put your body into this position and breathe fully. Allow your shoulders to drop and pull slightly back. Expand your chest a little.

Keep your spine erect but flexible. Walk tall.

In order to develop self-esteem we must give ourselves permission to think well of ourselves and to be successful. If we have grown up in a toxic or negative environment where it was not ok to "shine" we need to really challenge the value of this old view. We need to start to believe that it is ok to be ok. It is healthy to think well of yourself. It is fine to shine!

1. Having opened the door to the possibility of self-esteem we need to stop blocking affirmation and compliments. Using breathing technique we need to drink in actual compliments as they are delivered to us and to allow them to sit in our heart. Also, reflect on old compliments and breathe them down into your heart.

2. Allowing the affirmation or compliment houseroom is the first step the next step is to store them somewhere special. Using an actual or visualised receptacle place the compliment or affirmation in your receptacle. At times of difficulty or when you feel low return to your receptacle and remind yourself that people think well of you and love you. Remember that you are lovable.

Self Esteem: Generating Compassion & Kindness

3. If one compliment seems a flimsy basis for self-esteem remember how all the feathers of affirmation create a strong and supportive pillow or duvet to wrap around you!

4. Further techniques we can use to create compassion are to imagine someone or something we love, to feel the physical sensations of this and then project this love at ourselves. Also, meditating on accepting ourselves exactly where and how we are is a deepening of the first exercise.

5. If anger and hurt block us from developing compassion for ourselves then we need to follow the 6 stage programme:

6.

- Express this hurt by writing a letter to the person(s) who originally caused the pain.

- Develop the voice of a caring kind parent and decide to stop yearning for love or affirmation from someone who cannot give it

- Allow yourself time to let go of this yearning and grieve your loss

- Forgive and accept that your parents have limitations

- Clear your inner space to be able to generate compassion for yourself

- Find the love you need from people other than those who you insist "should" give you love.

Self Esteem: Generating Compassion & Kindness

Summary

This chapter has consisted mainly of exercises:

- Generating Love
- The Inner Mounting Flame
- Depth Acceptance
- Self Esteem & Anger
- The Kind Parent
- Grieving the Love You Wanted
- Forgiveness & Acceptance
- Clearing the Space for Love
- Finding the Love You Need
- The Self Esteem Smoothie
- The Self Esteem Treasure Chest
- Feathers & Pillows
- Physical Self Esteem

Chapter 11
Recovery & Renewal
The Programme

Introduction

In this book we have explored many ideas and now it is time to consider how we might draw all these components into a programme to help support you. This requires understanding three elements:

- The Key Concepts of Love Myself Slim

- Your Emotional Blueprint ie the patterns/rules which cause you to inhibit the expression of who you authentically are.

- The Exercises and practises which will best support you. Developing a daily and weekly programme to support your particular personality.

The Renewal and Recovery Programme

Key Concepts

Over-eating occurs primarily because we experience difficulty in expressing our emotions. This leads to a sense of frustration and emptiness. We "treat" these feelings by over-eating. To address the root cause of over-eating requires that we become more emotionally aware and emotionally expressive.

Our difficulties arises because:

The family rules we learnt about emotions taught us to inhibit emotional expression.

We were not taught to respect and value our own unique internal world of sensations, emotions, images and needs. This led to us dis-connecting from our bodies and minds which in turn creates the sense of emptiness and frustration.

- We did not experience sufficient compassion and acceptance as children. We may have received varying degrees of criticism or negativity. We therefore have learnt to be internally critical and lack kindness and compassion towards ourselves. We have frequently created a Critical Internal Voice. Rather than love ourselves as we are, we demand that we be different. This again leads to emptiness and frustration.

- We may frequently have been taught that everyone else's needs come first and that our own needs are secondary, irrelevant or downright stupid!

The Love Myself Slim programme seeks to raise awareness and actively start to reverse much of the emotional damage created by the ways of thinking outlined above. We need to create a four stage programme:

The Renewal and Recovery Programme

Stage One: Diagnosis:

On the basis of reflection and the use of exercises in this book we have analysed what has caused us to inhibit or limit our emotional expression. Even if we feel that we are quite emotionally expressive or even possibly volatile we need to explore why this does not meet our underlying emotional needs.

Find the Diagnostic Exercises listed in Appendix 1

Diagnosis requires that you understand the following information:

- What were the main rules which formed you regarding: Your body, food, emotions, control re. food, your position in the family, perfectionism. If you are struggling with this make a list of "shoulds" –see Excercise 2.8. This is a quick way to access your main "rules".

- Notice how the old family rules become internalised as a current Internal Critic or what I have called Self Talk. Notice how much in any given day you criticise or run a negative commentary on what you think or do.

- Contact Patterns: Projecting Emotion, Suppressing Emotion , Merging Identity, Self-Observing -how much are you practising any of the patterns detailed in the early chapters. Developing a better awareness of them will in itself help you change these patterns.

- Using the section on shame become aware of how shame -based you are. This will include understanding the degree to which you hide or bury your own needs.

- Carry out a needs review. What do you need to be happy and healthy.

The Renewal and Recovery Programme

- Notice how you eat and what this says about your approach to the world.

- Understand which particular thinking patterns trap you into particular ways of viewing yourself and the world.

- Using the Yes-No exercise discover what capacity, or not, you have for creating clear boundaries

Stage Two: How Can I Change?

Having recognised some of the emotional rules by which I have been operating I need to decide if I want to change any of this and if so how I will do this? Change can only begin by accepting where I am and then looking at what needs to be different. A major hurdle to change is often an inability to accept what "is", for example, that, "my father is really emotionally uncommunicative" or that "my mother is always critical of things I do". If I go on dreaming that "one day they will be different" – this will be a major impediment to my ability to change because I make it dependent upon someone else changing. This is VERY unlikely to happen!

Another impediment to change can be trying to take too big a step and then, having failed, believing change is not possible. After my angioplasty I kept over-exercising, making myself ill and then believing recovery was not possible, until I woke up to the fact that, for a while, I had to slow down. Then I got better!

For change to occur I have to decide I have had enough of the old ways and generate the courage to try small different steps. Many people scare themselves that the change they want is so difficult that it is impossible. With the help of the book and talking to friends or professionals create new words and phrases that you can first rehearse and then use when you wish to adopt a new approach. If change seems too difficult then it may either not be the right time to do this or you need to increase the level of support you have either from friends or professionals.

Change requires that you understand the following key idea:

You cannot begin a journey from London to Manchester by starting in Bristol. You have to begin any change process by starting exactly where you are! This means accepting who and how you are. Change does not occur by becoming someone different but rather by accepting and growing into who you truly are. All the meditation exercises can be helpful with this as well as Ex 9.1 Body Zones Awareness, Ex 10.3 Depth Acceptance, 10.1 Generating Love and Ex. 10.2 The Inner Mounting Flame which helps to develop a sense of value. Find a full list of these exercises in Appendix 1.

Stage Three: Expression & Discrimination

As has been described in some detail in the book once we have identified rules or behaviours which we were taught or received we need to find a positive way to express this. We can speak to the imaginary people or person concerned, we can write a letter we do not send or one of many other approaches outlined. If we are already expressive we need to check if what we are expressing is anger or rage which covers our sense of disappointment or hurt. If we feel angry it is important not only to find a way to express the anger but to let out our sense of hurt and pain.

Having expelled the anger and hurt from our system it is time to decide what sort of rules we want to live by and how we might start to be more compassionate and caring towards ourselves. Discrimination requires that we go back through our family history and sift and sort what was emotionally or psychologically useful and what we need to let go of. Ensuring that we have fully expressed the hurt or pain we can then start to re-build who or how we want to be.

If we imagine that old emotional pain is like a blockage in what should be a free-flowing stream of feeling then expression is a form of psycho-Dynarod. Expression does not have to be necessarily dramatic or angry although it can be. Rather, it entails a real commitment to deciding that the old way is no longer useful. It is therefore important to give back whatever you received which was not useful. Only by doing this can you clear your emotional-energetic system and make space for something better and more loving.

Using the Expression Exercises in Appendix 1 you can explore a wide variety of ways to start with this. Only do what feels safe and comfortable enough. I urge caution with clients who want to directly express something, particularly anger and aggression, to another person. A client who recently became very angry with her brother was going to "completely end the relationship, forever". I pointed out that "forever" is a very long time! Two weeks later she gave up on the idea. It was enough to simply express her anger and frustration with him. Writing a letter you do not send can often be more freeing than one which you do.

Stage Four: Your New Identity: Commitment, Support & Application

Creating a new identity or sense of self can be a challenging and scary business. What it most requires is both commitment to the "new you" and the application of the exercises and homework suggested. Developing improved Internal and External Support is the key to the new you!

The Renewal and Recovery Programme

Your Programme

As human beings we are all unique and have our own history and our own way of being. Whilst trying all the exercises you will no doubt find more use and benefit in some rather than others. Build your own programme from the exercises you find most helpful.

To get the most from this programme you need to commit some regular time to the exercises. Making time may well be your first challenge. All I can say is that if you continue to do the same things you will get the same results! You will get the most from this programme if you mix up the exercises which challenge you along with some that support you.

So, start with the Diagnostic exercises. Try to work out what your core family rules are and then start to give back the ones which are no longer useful to you. This will move you into the Expressive Exercises. Continue working through the Diagnostic exercises moving into the Expressive Exercises as you need to let go of elements of your past. Using the Expressive Exercises try to develop a more emotionally expressive style that supports you from bottling up new difficulties. Remember to listen to your body and sensations to understand what your needs are. Become more expressive about articulating these needs whilst balancing compassion and consideration for others. Ensure though that sufficient of your core needs are being met.

The Meditation Exercises can be started immediately and run in parallel with the others. Sitting and stilling your mind in the ways described can be very beneficial. Start with Meditating on the 10 Zones, follow this with Meditation on The Breath and finally the Meditation on the Body. Initially, try sitting for just 5 -10 mins using one of the foci described. As you develop your ability, sit for longer. The mp3 tracks

The Renewal and Recovery Programme

(available at www.dialogueconsultancy.com) are there to assist you in these meditations. As you develop though you may want to try meditating without this help, simply sitting with yourself. The Micro-Meditation can be introduced after a few weeks of practice. This will also help consolidate you in living and working more from a place of "Being" rather than just "Doing".

Love Myself Slim & Dieting

You may have wondered why there is no mention of diets in a book on over-eating. This is because I strongly believe that if you do not address your own psychology then whatever your diet plan you are likely to fail. We are all unique and may require differing amounts of time to complete the programme. One of my clients, who was very over-weight, spent a year working through the Love Myself Slim plan. At the end of the year she started a diet and has been highly successful in losing a lot of weight. From the outset though the aim was to deal with the under-lying issues. Once these were resolved her diet was simply the cherry on the cake – if you'll excuse a culinary analogy! At the end of the process she is far happier, more confident AND much slimmer!

Another client who was bingeing and vomiting up to 5 times a day followed the plan for a month with dramatic changes occurring almost as soon as she understood the connection between emotional expression and her eating patterns. She has now returned to a far more normal eating pattern and no longer vomits.

Developing an emotionally expressive and communicative approach to life can rapidly produce change. Combining this with a more mindful approach to ourselves and our eating can fully support this change.

The Renewal and Recovery Programme

I have tried in this book to give you all the elements which I know can make a big diference to the way you function in yourself with and around food. However, only you can finally pull this into a package which really works for you. Explore the book and then map out a programme of what you need to work on and which exercises you feel will most support you. Good luck!

The Renewal and Recovery Programme

APPENDIX 1

	1. DIAGNOSTIC EXERCISES	
1.1	Body & Emotions	Notice how your body opens and closes to positive & negative thoughts
1.2	Body Zones Introduction	Become aware of the sensations in your body. Learn to listen more carefully to the data from your body
2.1	Body Rules	What family rules were there about your body and how to relate to it
2.2	Food Rules	What family rules were there regarding food. What did food mean in your family?
2.3	Family Position	What position do you hold in your family and what significance does that have
2.5	Approval	Explore the degree to which your value is based upon the approval of your family

The Renewal and Recovery Programme

2.8	"Shoulds"	Very important. Listing "shoulds" will reveal unexamined rules from childhood. It's time to find out what they are and whether you need to still adhere to them
2.12	The Yes-No Game	Very important. This exercise reveals how easy or otherwise it is to say No. Also, how you can support yourself to become better at assertion.
3.1	Rules About Emotions	What family rules were there regarding the expression of emotions
3.2	Top Rules About Emotions	What were the most important family rules about the expression of emotions
3.3	Family Rules & Self Talk	How do the family rules around emotion and criticism generally become internalised as "Self Talk"?
3.6	Perfectionism	How do you set yourself up to be perfect?

The Renewal and Recovery Programme

3.7	Impulse Control	Learning to slow down your response to feeling empty, frustrated or unhappy so that you do not over-react or over-eat
3.8	"Sitting on Things"	What happens when you do not express how you feel?
4.6	Needs Review	What are your essential needs to feel happy and healthy?
5.1	Projection	What is projection and how do you project onto other people?
5.2	Self-Observing	Exploring your capacity to self observe
7.1	Shame & Contempt	How contempt can cover and mask te experience of shame
7.2	Shame & Envy	How envy can cover and mask the experience of shame
7.3	Anger & Irritability	How anger and irritability can cover and mask the experience of shame.
7.4	Shame Questionnaire	How shame-based are you? Complete the questionnaire

The Renewal and Recovery Programme

7.5	How Shame Arises	Explore how shame may develop and arise in you
7.6	Unacceptable Needs	Explore what needs were unacceptable in your family
8.1	How You Eat	Observing carefully how you eat and what this says about you.
8.3	Needs & Difference	Exploring your needs and your acceptance of your difference
8.4	Food & Control	What were the family rules around food as a mechanism for control.
9.5	Fantasy & Fact	Distinguishing between fantasy and fact
9.6	Thinking Traps	Learn the thinking patterns you trap you into particular ways of viewing yourself and the world
9.7	Pleasant Unpleasant experiences	Exploring the meaning you make of pleasant and unpleasant experiences

The Renewal and Recovery Programme

	EXERCISES PARTICULARLY FOCUSSING ON CHANGE AS SELF ACCEPTANCE	
8.2	Eating Mindfully	Eating slowly and mindfully can be a real challenge & support to allowing yourself to be with yourself.
8.3	Needs & Difference	Can you have different needs to other people and be ok?
9.1	Body Zones Awareness	Simply sitting with yourself, breathing fully and being with your body is a first step in self-acceptance
9.3	Mindfull Breathing	Being with yourself & breathing consciously is a second step in self-acceptance
9.4	The Full Mindful Breath	This exercise can be hugely supportive. Practice every day for a fortnight and then use whenever you feel anxious or stressed. It **will** make a difference!
10.1	Generating Love	This exercise challenges you to offer the same degree of love to yourself as to a person or animal which is close to you.

The Renewal and Recovery Programme

10.2	The Inner Mounting Flame	Developing a clear visual representation of your unwavering self-acceptance can help support your development of self-esteem
10.3	Depth Acceptance	Change requires a deep acceptance of who and how we are. This exercise encourages and supports this approach.
10.6	Grieving the Love You Wanted	Letting go of our fantasy of the love we might have had is a major step in starting to love ourselves in the here-and-now
10.7	Forgiveness & Acceptance	Forgiving yourself and others is again a crucial way to allow yourself to live in the present with more compassion and acceptance

	3. EXPRESSION EXERCISES	
2.4	Expressing Emotion about an Old Rule	Re-connecting with how you felt about the imposition of an old family rule can help you to begin to understand if this is still a rule you wish to live by.

The Renewal and Recovery Programme

2.6	Confluence	Beginning to understand and break the confluence will enable you to grow enormously in your own sense of value
2.7	Challenging the Lock-In	You can love people and still not agree with them. Blindly accepting a "truth" is not healthy or helpful
2.9	Aggressive Internalised Parent	This can take a lot of courage but standing up to your internalised parent can produce huge changes in your sense of self-value and boundary -making. Always ensure you feel sufficiently supported to do this exercise.
2.11	Emotionally Manipulative Internalised Parent	Emotional manipulation can be as damaging if not more so than a parent who is directly aggressive. Again, this can help you to find your sense of value and of appropriate boundary-making
2.12	"I am Your Equal"	Remembering you are equal and expressing it to yourself and manifesting it in your behaviour will start to rectify the imbalance of feeling less than.

The Renewal and Recovery Programme

2.12	Saying "No"	Practicing saying "No" will enable you to set boundaries and limitations and to start living more authentically
2.14	Closure	What is unfinished continues to loop around inside us both emotionally and cognitively. Closure stops this.
3.4	Letter to Your Parents	Expressing what your experience of being a child was like and how you need to move forward positively with your own distinct identity
3.5	Self Support & Self-Expression	Improving your awareness of how to support yourself and to express who you are
4.4	Being Authentic	Exploring expressing more of what you truly feel moving away from what Fritz Perls called The Cliche Layer!

4.5	Authenticity & Compassion	Practising authenticity with compassion
10.4	Expressing Hurt & Anger	Expressing the pain and hurt that is underneath your anger

4. COMMITMENT, SUPPORT & APPLICATION		
3.6	Perfectionism	Explore your perfectionism and find ways to be less demanding of yourself – and others
3.7	Impulse Control	Move out of "automatic" and discover what you really need
4.1	Humour	When humour acts as defence to authenticity or shame
4.2	Silence	Exploring silence

The Renewal and Recovery Programme

4.3	Being Alone	Discover what being alone means to you
4.4	Being Authentic	Improving your awareness of how to support yourself and to express who you are
5.3	Affirmation & Breathing	Breathing affirmations through your body
5.4	Inner- Outer & Middle Zones	Understanding the different Zones of functioning
6.1	Tuning into Sensation	Becoming even more aware of your body and it's responses
6.2	Inner Zone	Living from your felt-sense of reality rather than the fantasy of the Middle Zone
6.3	Sensation-Image-Though-Feeling	Understanding how emotion is grounded in sensation

The Renewal and Recovery Programme

7.7	Developing a Positive Internal Voice	Change your Self Talk from negative to positive

9.2	Eating Mindfully	Eating slowly and mindfully can be a real challenge & support to allowing yourself to be with yourself.
9.3	Mindful Breathing	Being with yourself & breathing consciously is a second step in self-acceptance
9.4	The Full Mindful Breath	This exercise can be hugely supportive. Practice every day for a fortnight and then use whenever you feel anxious or stressed. It will make a difference!
9.8	Meditating on the Body	Expanding your awareness from a breath focus to a body focus can enable your meditation to go to a deeper level of calm relaxed energy.
9.9	The Micro-Meditation	Practising Micro-Meditations even if for only 2 -3 minutes during the day can help calm and energise you.

The Renewal and Recovery Programme

10.1	Generating Love	This exercise challenges you to offer the same degree of love to yourself as to a person or an animal to which you are close
10.2	The Inner Mounting Flame	Developing a clear visual representation of your unwavering self-acceptance can help support your development of self-esteem
10.3	Depth Acceptance	Change requires a deep acceptance of who and how we are. This exercise encourages and supports this approach.
10.5	The Kind Parent	Developing a kinder internal voice by using the voice you would use as a parent. i.e being re-assuring, calming and encouraging
10.9	Finding the Love you Need	Having started to let go of looking for your fantasy of love start loving yourself more but also develop friendships which are loving and positive.

The Renewal and Recovery Programme

Chapter Notes ...see Bibliography for full details

Chapter 3

P.44 Gerhardt, S *Why Love Matters*

P.45 Cozolino L *The Neuroscience of Psychotherapy*

Chapter 5

P.**96** Perls, F *Gestalt Therapy*

Chapter 6

P.105 Gladwell M(2007) *Blink*

Chapter 7

P113 Yontef, G *Awareness, Dialogue and Process*

P.122 Mackewn,J *Developing Gestalt Counselling.*

Chapter 8

P134 Perls, F *Gestalt Therapy* .

P.136 Perls F *Gestalt Therapy*

Chapter 9

P.142 Kabat Zinn) *Full Catastrophe Living*

P.142 Frankl,V *Man's Search for Meaning*

Chapter 10

Gilbert,P *Compassion*

The Renewal and Recovery Programme

Bibliography & Resources

Books on Gestalt

Joyce, P and Sills,C (2010): *Skills in Gestalt Counselling & Psychotherapy*. London Sage

An excellent introduction to contemporary Gestalt Therapy

Mackewn, J(1997) *Developing Gestalt Counselling*. London. Sage

Another excellent introduction to contemporary Gestalt Therapy

Perls,F, Hefferline,R, Goodman (1951) *Gestalt Therapy..* London. Souvenir Press

The original bible of Gestalt Therapy from Fritz Perls et al. Demanding yet rewarding reading if you really want to understand what Gestalt is about.

Yontef, G *Awareness, Dialogue and Process*. Gestalt Journal Press,U.S. (1 July 1993)

Contemporary refining of the original teaching of Gestalt

Books on Mindfulness

Kabbatt-Zinn J(1990) *Full Catastrophe Living*. London. Piatkus plus many other titles by this author.

If you wish to read about the practice of contemporary Mindfulness this is the place to start. Kabat-Zinn is the man who brought a secular version of Buddhism into mainstream mental health practice.

The Renewal and Recovery Programme

Books on Neuroscience & or Compassion

Gerhardt, S (2004) *Why Love Matters*. Routledge

Compelling read. How affection shapes the development of the baby's brain

Gilbert, P.(2009) *The Compassionate Mind. London.* Constable

Describes the impact of compassion upon the development of the brain and generally upon mental health.

Cozolino, L . *The Neuroscience of Psychotherapy.*

Excellent academic tome on the interface between neuroscience and Psychotherapy. Very readable.

Books on Shame

Bradshaw J.(20006) *Healing The Shame That Binds You.*

Publisher: Health Communications

Great classic on working with issues of shame

Existential

Frankl,V. Man's Search for Meaning. Rider & Co; New edition edition (2004)

Existential classic

General

Gladwell,M(2007) *Blink Back Bay Books*

How and why you should trust your intuitive response

The Renewal and Recovery Programme

Breathing & Meditation Exercises

All exercises are available as free downloadable mp3 tracks at www.dialogueconsultancy.com comments or enquiries to jonathan@dialogueconsultancy.com. The current tracks are:

1. The Ten Zones
2. The Full Mindful Breath
3. Meditating on your Breath
4. Meditating on Your Body
5. Meditating on Sound
6. Micro-Meditation

The Renewal and Recovery Programme

Glossary

This book has been written for a general readership. As such I have edited out most technical psychotherapy language to hopefully make the book more user friendly. However some readers who have an understanding of therapy, especially Gestalt therapy, may have recognised many of the ideas but wondered to which element of Gestalt terminology I was referring. Equally, for readers who may be interested in deepening their understanding of the wonderful and fascinating realm of contemporary Gestalt it may be useful to learn a little of the language of Gestalt.

In the earlier chapters of the book I discuss how we block or interrupt emotional contact with ourselves in various ways. There are a number of technical terms which I will describe:

De-sensitisation: We learn to de-sensitise by disconnecting from the somatic information from our body. A classic example of this was a nurse in a workshop on stress who in response to "How do you know when to eat?" said " I eat because it's one o clock!". She had little or no awareness of her body because she was so used to over-working and putting her patients first. I refer in the book to de-sensitisation as " Blanking".

Confluence: Confluence arises when our identity becomes merged – usually with one or both parents. We are expected to accord with their wishes. If we do not, love or acceptance is withdrawn. The child is then faced with the dilemma of being true to themselves and being rejected or going along with what their parents want but giving up on some element of themselves.

Most children want the love and acceptance and forego themselves. In the book I refer to this as "Identity Merger".

The Renewal and Recovery Programme

Introjection: Is the process whereby I take on the rules of my family. Introjected rules are usually seen as rules which have been unquestioningly swallowed down. Perls, makes the parallel with a piece of food being swallowed whole and not chewed and properly assimilated. To lead a more conscious and aware life we need to "chew over" the rules we were given as children and decide if they are something we still wish to lead our lives by. In the book I refer to introjects simply as "Rules".

Retroflection: Is the process whereby I suppress my anger, rage or simply my reaction. If something unpleasant occurs our natural response is to become angry, to react. If as children we are repeatedly taught that it is not ok to express our reactions then we learn to retroflect or suppress our emotions. Clearly, there are times when it is important to control our emotions but if suppression becomes a generalised response to feeling emotions then we become what is known as, retroflected ie we hold in our emotion. As the book describes retroflection is a major element in over-eating. In the book I generally refer to this process as "suppressing emotion".

Projection: Occurs when we dump a disowned emotion of our own on someone else. We might feel angry with a friend because they have a better job than us but then criticise the friend for being arrogant or self-important. We "project" our envy onto them and make them bad rather than being able to own that we wish we had such

a great job! In the book I use the word projection but also talk about "putting our emotions onto others".

Egotising: Occurs when we slightly dis-engage from ourselves and watch ourselves or run a commentary, usually critical, upon what we do. This leads to a self-conscious, somewhat disconnected way of functioning which lacks spontaneity. In the book I describe this as "self-observing".

The Renewal and Recovery Programme

The Renewal and Recovery Programme

Index

A

Acknowledgements 6
Affirmation 108
Anger & Irritability 131
Anger & Shame
  Ex 132
Approval 28
  Ex 29
Assertion 79
Authenticity and Compassion 93
Authentic vs In-authentic 91
Awareness
  interrupting cycle 15
Awareness,Cycle 12

B

Barriers to Meditation 176
Being Alone 89
  Ex 90
Being Authentic!
  Ex 92
Bibliography & Resources 217
Blanking 117
Body 9
  rules 16
  Rules Ex 17
  Zones Ex 10
Body Zones Awareness
  Ex 158
Breathing & Meditation Exercises 219

The Renewal and Recovery Programme

C

Caring cinderella 67, 70
Change 198

Chapter Notes 215
Closure 53
  Ex 54
Compassion & Self-Esteem 179
Compliments, blocking 189
Conflict- avaoidance 46
Confluence 32, 220
Contact 7
Cycle of Awareness 74

D

Defensiveness 102
Depth Acceptance 183
De-sensitisation 220
De-Sensitising 117
Diagnosis 197
Diagnostic Exercises 204
Dieting 202
Diets 1
Doing & Being Mode 85

E

Eating
  how you 149
Eating Mindfully
  Ex 150, 160
Egotising 221
Emotion
  and control mechanisms 65
  suppressing 80
  suppressing with food 62

The Renewal and Recovery Programme

Emotional Blueprint 195
Emotions
  and family rules 59
Equality 44
  Ex 45
Expressing emotion 24
Expressing Hurt & Anger 185
Expression & Discrimination 199
Eye Contact 89

F

Family Position 20–57
  Ex 23
  rules 20
Family rules
  and self talk 65
Family rules about emotions Ex 60
Fantasy & Fact
  Ex 166
Fantasy vs reality 29
Feathers & Pillows
  Ex 191
Feelings
  avoiding 84
Food
  and meaning 153
  control and 154
  rules 17
  rules Ex 19
Forgiveness & Acceptance
  Ex 187

G

Generating Love
  Ex 181
Globalising vs discriminating 29
Glossary 220

H

Here & Now 109, 157

I

Identity 7
  development 148
Identity and contact 7
Impulse Control
  Ex 76
Impulsivity 73
Inner Mounting Flame
  Ex 182
Inner Zone
  Ex 120
Introjection 221

K

Key Concepts 195, 196

L

Letter to...
  your parenrs 67
Lock-in 32
  challenging Ex 34
Love
  and grieving 186
  clearing a space for
    Ex 187
  finding it Ex 188
Love, and affection 58

M

Meditating on Your Body 172
Merging 30
  identity, Ex 32

The Renewal and Recovery Programme

Micro-Meditation 173
Mindful Breathing
  Ex 161

Mindfulness & Over-eating 156

N

Needs & Difference
  Ex 152
Needs Review 96

O

Over-eating
  a psychological profile 54

P

Parent, historic vs actual 27
Parents
  aggressive 39
  manipulative 43
Parent, the kind 186
Perfectionism
  Ex 72
Perfect Princess 71
Pleasant & Unpleasant Experiences 169
POWER 104
Programme, your 201
Projection 100, 221
  Ex 101
Projection & Over-Eating 103

R

Recovery & Renewal 195
Retroflection 221
Rule
  checklist 26

The Renewal and Recovery Programme

Rules
  about you 19

S

Self Esteem
  physical 192
Self-Esteem & Anger 184
Self Esteem Smoothie 189
Self-Esteem Treasure Chest 191
Self-support
  improving 68
Self talk 66
Sensation 8, 118
  image-thought-feeling 125
Sensations to Needs 123
Shaame 127
Shame
  contempt and 130
  defending against 130
  envy, and 131
  how it arises 136
  how it is expressed 129
  internalising of 139
  management 145
  re. being over-weight 145
  recovery from 141
Shame Binds 138
Shame Questionnaire 133
Shoulds, Ex 37
Silence 88
Support
  internal...external 69

T

The Full Mindful Breath
  Ex 164

The Renewal and Recovery Programme

Thinking Traps 168

W
Watching Yourself 107

Y

Yes-No Game Ex 47
Your Programme 201

Z

Zones,three 110
   Ex 112